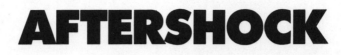

AFTERSHOCK

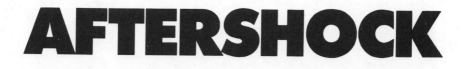

AFTERSHOCK

Surviving the Delayed Effects of
Trauma, Crisis and Loss

ANDREW E. SLABY, M.D., PH.D., M.P.H.

VILLARD BOOKS · NEW YORK · 1989

Grateful acknowledgment is made to the following for permission to reprint previously published material:

American Health: Excerpts from "How Much Stress Can You
Survive?" *American Health* magazine © 1984. Reprinted by
permission.

Newsweek: Excerpt from "Ten Tough Jobs" from *Newsweek*,
April 25, 1988. Copyright © 1988 by Newsweek, Inc. All rights
reserved. Used by permission.

Library of Congress Cataloging-in-Publication Data
Slaby, Andrew Edmund.
    Aftershock: surviving the delayed effects of trauma, crisis
and loss.
    1. Posttraumatic stress disorder—Popular works.
I. Title.
RC552.P67S57   1989   616.85′21   88-27687
ISBN 0-394-57403-6

Although the case histories in this book are accurate, the
names and identifying characteristics of the persons described
have been changed to protect their privacy.

Manufactured in the United States of America
9 8 7 6 5 4 3 2
First Edition

Produced by P.I.A. Specialty Press, Inc.
Designer: Stephanie Bart-Horvath

To my parents, Andrew and Evelyn Herde Slaby,
and to
Victoria Ehrhardt Morse

ACKNOWLEDGMENTS

THIS BOOK, LIKE ALL BOOKS, REPRESENTS A STATEMENT not from the author alone, but from all who have contributed to its content and form. In particular, Dr. Arvin Glicksman, Professor of Radiation Biology at Brown, is acknowledged for his previous work with me on life-threatening illness. This work, published in *Adapting to Life-Threatening Illness* (New York: Praeger Press, 1985), is discussed extensively in a number of places throughout the book.

I am especially grateful to Karla Dougherty, whose considerable talents made invaluable contributions to the book's writing and research. And to Larry Chilnick and Dan Montopoli, whose efforts made this book possible.

To all of these people, I extend my special gratitude.

C O N T E N T S

PART THREE: AFTERSHOCK THERAPY

PART FOUR: LIVING WELL AND HAPPY IN A SHOCKING WORLD

INTRODUCTION

AFTERSHOCK—GROWTH THROUGH CRISIS

> *The best way out is always through.*
> —HELEN KELLER

You walk to work the same way, the same time, every day. This one day, however, on the walk to work you hear a noise. You look up as you see your neighbor stumbling out of his house. As he falls, you notice there's blood everywhere, half his face is missing. You freeze. You want to run away but you can't—there are children on their way to school and they've seen him too. You go over to help him, not knowing what to do. He says over and over again, "Leave me alone, leave me alone." You go inside and call an ambulance. You try to cover his face with your coat but he throws the coat away, saying "Let me die. Please, let me die." The ambulance comes and he fights with the attendants. Finally they take him away. You go home and you throw up. You realize you never even knew the man's first name. You never talk to anybody about what happened. But for the last twenty years there hasn't been a day when you didn't think about that guy, when his words didn't haunt you. You wish that day never happened.

As A PSYCHIATRIST SPECIALIZING IN CRISIS THERAPY and prevention, I have helped hundreds of patients cope with the entire realm of human experience. I have heard stories of incredible pain and incredible strength. I've seen the effects of a crisis firsthand in men and women suffering from cancer, in combat veterans home from Vietnam, in accident victims and crime victims, in children who have felt the pangs of divorce, in anorexic teenagers, and in countless others—each of them unique, but at the same time each sharing in the universal trials and tribulations inherent in everyday living. The resiliency, strength, and determination of the human race to survive in the face of overwhelming obstacles provides all of us with inspiration.

Yet, there are times when our best defenses prove inadequate, when all the tricks and strategies we have learned simply are not enough and we feel powerless, with seemingly no recourse but to rail against the unfairness of life and to wish for better times.

If wishes were reality, we would all be rich, good looking, young, and carefree. There would be no upsets, no downswings, and no fears or anxieties to keep us up at night. Like characters in a fairy tale, we would whisk away our hardships by rubbing a magic lamp or wishing on the first evening star.

The idea of "happily ever after" might be the stuff of make-believe, but its underlying desire is very real and very resilient. Whether we use yesterday's magic or today's power of positive thinking, we still want a direct line to health, happiness, and success in our everyday lives.

And why not? From movies and magazines to books and prime-time TV, the world is ready to dazzle us with the proof that everything we want is within our grasp—*if* we stay fit and healthy, *if* we eat and drink sensibly, *if* we manage to maintain a positive, confident attitude. "Go for it!" is the slogan of our times.

But the fact is that we sometimes can't go for it. Real life is a constantly changing road—some of it predictable, some of it totally out of our control. We can certainly help things along by eating right and living right, but that won't prevent a major flood or the death of a loved one. Despite our best intentions, we may still get fired from our job. With or without our consent, sunny skies can become stormy, the stock market can go haywire, and the kindest people can come to harm.

When things change suddenly, they can shake up our world, sometimes with painful results that come back to destroy our emotional equilibrium long after the traumatic events themselves have passed.

THAT'S LIFE

"It isn't fair!"

"I'm in shock. I never expected to win!"

"I don't believe this is happening to me."

"I saw it with my own eyes!"

"I am so afraid it will happen again."

"I feel so all alone."

"It's everything I ever wanted. So why do I feel so bad?"

Events that change our lives are traumatic in any guise. Whether it's moving to an exciting new home in a distant city or a wrenching personal tragedy, such an event can affect us heart and soul. A life-changing event is made even more startling in today's fast-paced world, where there is so little time to absorb what's happening and where we tend to put aside our feelings, carry on as usual, and keep our emotions to ourselves. We admire a stiff upper lip as a positive, confident sign of our strength. Witness the world's response to Jackie Kennedy as she stood tall at her husband's funeral. As JFK was lowered into the ground, she moved not a muscle on her face, a study of composure and poise.

What the public doesn't see, however, is the suffering that can strike weeks, months, and years after the traumatic event. While serving as Director of Emergency Services at Yale–New Haven Hospital, I confronted one very complex case that illustrates how insidious this suffering can be.

A certain Mr. Williams had been playing a doubles handball match with his three sons every Saturday for almost fifteen years. Williams, now in his late fifties and a very successful senior law partner with a prominent law firm, cherished these weekly get-togethers. As you might expect, his sons were a little more ambivalent. While they usually enjoyed these occasions, there were times when they would be delayed or simply could not fit the game into their schedules. At such times they resented the matches.

One Saturday each son independently of the other called his father to tell him they would be late. Instead of waiting for his sons, Williams decided to play a singles match instead. During the game he suffered a fatal heart attack. As each son arrived at the health club, he was confronted with the shocking news: his father, who had never spent even one night in a hospital, was dead.

Six months pass. The eldest son, who until his father's death was a very successful vice president of a major corporation, had simply stopped going to work. On the verge of losing his job, he spent most of his time at home while his employees scrambled to cover for his absence. The second son, a professor at a prestigious Eastern college, now insisted on starting his own family. Unfortunately, his wife had no desire to interrupt her own career at this time. Unable to resolve their differences, the couple had begun to drift apart. The third son, having just been named a junior partner at his father's old law firm, began working incredibly long hours, driving up his billable time, while ignoring his personal life. Recently his fiancée had postponed their wedding indefinitely.

All of the sons were suffering from a condition that I call *aftershock.*

Many of us have had aftershock experiences, going through the first stages of a crisis numb and in shock, only to wake up one morning a few days, weeks, or even months later in tears, the full impact of what happened finally hitting home.

A few people may be so traumatized by a crisis that they actually find themselves overresponding both physically and mentally to a sight, a sound, or a smell that reminds them of the original event, sometimes to the point where they relive the original experience in frightening and realistic detail. This response is called *posttraumatic stress disorder (PTSD)* and it is a major element of aftershock. But aftershock is more than PTSD. In my practice, I coined the term *"aftershock"* to describe any significant delayed response to a crisis, whether this reaction is anxiety, depression, substance abuse, or PTSD.

In counseling patients, I have found that explaining this delayed reaction as an aftershock helps them to better understand their situation. I usually tell them that aftershock is a term borrowed from geology, where it is used to describe the rebound tremor that follows an earthquake. Often it is the aftershock—by striking already weakened structures—that does the most damage, not the initial earthquake.

In humans it is lives, relationships, and careers, not buildings, that can be destroyed by aftershock. Left untreated and undetected, aftershock can create psychological and physical problems, from depression and sexual dysfunction to heart ailments and anxiety attacks. But help is at hand. Aftershock can be overcome. We might not be able to take away life's dramatic upheavals, but with understanding, we can learn to survive them, and perhaps most important, we can even learn to prepare ourselves to overcome these dramatic upheavals *before* they strike.

How many of us suffer from aftershock? Frankly, the hard numbers, even the reliable estimates that give us the illusion of having a handle on the problem, are simply not yet available. Whether it is because the symptoms of aftershock often resemble other psychiatric conditions, such as anxiety or depression, or because psychiatry in general has been slow to recognize PTSD as more than battle fatigue, the number of aftershock victims remains mysterious. However, I do believe that this lack of hard scientific data will not last. Hopefully, as psychiatry speeds toward the twenty-first century, aftershock will receive the full attention it deserves.

FINDING GROWTH, HEALTH, AND SERENITY IN TRYING TIMES

In 1918, Dr. Colin K. Russel said that the symptoms of aftershock were the natural reactions "of the mind in suppressing the unpleasant truth that he is afraid." This book will help you feel that fear, understand it, and strengthen your resolve to go on—happier, more fulfilled, and wiser. It will help you to identify and understand aftershock in yourself and in those around you. It can serve as a guide to curing aftershock and stopping it in its tracks and as a sourcebook for its prevention—via a hardier, more resilient personality that can better adapt to both life's setbacks and its successes.

The first part of *Aftershock* will help you recognize the syndrome in all its forms, from emotional turmoil to physical ailments. In addition, the book will explain the differences between aftershock and other psychiatric conditions such as general anxiety disorder, panic attacks, and depression. The second part pinpoints the traumas of the 1980s that can set off aftershock: events of global impact, personal crimes of the heart, and corporate games in today's business world. The third part details the exciting cures available today, both in pharmaceutical medicine and in psychiatry. And the fourth and final section teaches you ways to prevent aftershock and its aftermath from disrupting your world ever again.

Maybe there really is a life after death. Maybe we do get a second chance here on earth. We will never know; we only know and have the here and now. And understanding aftershock will help make the here and now the best it can be—for yourself and for those you love. And that's worth a lot.

PART ONE:

THE SHOCKING TRUTH

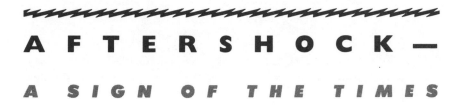

AFTERSHOCK—
A SIGN OF THE TIMES

FIVE . . . FOUR . . . THREE . . . TWO . . . ONE . . . Suddenly there are screams, shouts—and on the air, in front of our eyes, the space shuttle explodes into a fiery ball. All seven crew members, including teacher Christa McAuliffe are dead. The world is shocked. Millions are numb, unable to accept the tragedy. The space program is halted, its momentum lost. And school children no longer aspire to be astronauts when they grow up.

Rhoda is an attractive, seemingly healthy middle-aged woman, with a mysterious problem; she cannot leave her house. Not too long ago, she was a secure woman, happily married for the last thirty-one years to the man that she still loved. With her children grown and enjoying lives of their own, Rhoda was looking forward to her first visit to Europe with her husband. Then suddenly he comes home and tells her he wants a divorce. He loves her, but he doesn't want to live with her anymore. Rhoda is shocked; she can't believe it. At first she denies it, but after the smoke clears, after the lawyers have all had their say, she goes home—and is terrified to leave the house for even the simplest errands.

Richard is the golden boy of a Wall Street firm. Only twenty-five years old, he is making a six-figure salary and enjoying the good life with an expensive apartment, a fashionable car, and a promising future. Then the stock market plummets. People are out of work, including Richard. He was the golden boy; it shouldn't have happened to him. But it did. He tries to find another job, but there aren't any out there. To feel better, he starts to drink . . . and drink.

Margo and Tom have just had their first baby. It's a wonderful, healthy little boy. They call him Jason and Tom is enchanted with him. But Margo doesn't want anything to do with Jason; she can't hold him and she has become distant. Everyone calls it postpartum blues, but it's more than that. Margo's father died when she was just an infant. It's something she can barely recall. But somehow the shock of *then* has come out *now* with the joyous event of her own child's birth.

Robert, too, had cause for celebration. He had had a heart attack several years ago, but with the proper care he has fully recovered. At first he was afraid to go back to work, but eventually, as his good health continued, he was back on a normal routine. He did so well, in fact, that he received a promotion. Everything was on track again. But suddenly Robert started having imaginary chest pains. Suddenly he was afraid to go into the office. He felt himself slipping backward, and he just knew he was going to die.

These real-life scenarios are all examples of aftershock. Once, almost everyone assumed that aftershock was exclusively contracted during war, a result of battleground shell shock. And recently we have heard a lot about PTSD and Vietnam veterans. So much so, that the mention of PTSD conjures up a vision of a Rambo-like veteran dressed in camouflage, hurling his rifle from a mountain cliff back in the States, the war continuing in his own head—or of the veteran who went into a local McDonald's and killed twenty-one patrons. But these are the bigger-than-life examples, the terrifying horror stories that are the rare exceptions to the rules. Yes, these tortured vets did suffer from PTSD and aftershock, and yes, it was war that first brought this condition to our attention—but it's more than that.

We all suffer from aftershock, maybe less violently but still at a price we shouldn't have to pay. In fact, aftershock is the disease of today.

THE EIGHTIES FALLOUT

The "good old days" may never have been, but life long ago was very different. Things were done at leisure; it took longer to get news. In 1815, for example, it took three weeks to travel between New York and Cincinnati. Travel and commerce were so difficult that most Americans actually produced the goods that they themselves ate, wore, or otherwise used. Information traveled so slowly that the last major battle of the War of 1812, in which numerous soldiers died, was actually fought after the war had ended; the combatants did not know that peace had been declared. Today, we merely switch on our television or pick up the phone and we are instantly connected to the outside world.

Immediacy, instant replay, information please—none of these expressions existed in the past or mean what they mean now. The outside world was no bigger than the next village or the legendary Big City to which visits were as awesome as pilgrimages. Life centered on the family. Entire communities celebrated births and participated in deaths. With so much plague, disease, and ignorance, death was as commonplace and as expected as the coming of spring. People didn't try to prolong their lives; they couldn't. There were no exercise machines, fiber-rich diets, or pills that made you well. You lived, and then you died. Lady Antonia Fraser writes that aristocratic parents never bothered even to get close to their children until they were five years old, an age when their survival was more assured. Rich and poor alike had a great many children, so when one died, there would be others still at home.

Death was expected, as was one's role in life. If you were lucky enough to be born into money, you assumed you would have it forever. Kings ruled and subjects revered them. Men and women married and were expected to stay together until death, perhaps in a house that had been in the family for generations. Marriage, financial status, even the place where you were born and raised—all stayed the same; all was constant. This status quo gave people roots, a confidence that sprung from consistency, a security that their expectations would be met. And the family unit helped keep the hostile world at bay.

Not so today. Our families have divided, our communities have dissolved, and our hectic schedules leave little time to absorb the world around us.

Expectations, too, are more complicated in the 1980s. We expect more than just an existence anchored to the changing seasons, life and death, hearth and home. We expect to live longer. We expect to have our piece of the pie. We expect our children to have everything. And we expect to fall in love and marry if that's what we want.

Information brings knowledge and, with knowledge, we become more sophisticated. Because we have newspapers, magazines, television with its *Lifestyles of the Rich and Famous*, we learn what otherwise might be beyond our imagination. We can see and read about the products that promise success. We can also see the crime, the hopelessness, and the violence—all assimilated within minutes on the same TV show.

We live today under the constant threat of nuclear holocaust and under an avalanche of illegal drugs that threatens to destroy our cities and the lives of our children. At no time in our history has the threat to all human life been as great as it is today. And we must face these increasingly greater pressures with an ever-increasing divorce rate, and with the dissolution of our extended families.

But still we absorb the information. And we still yearn for something better. We still want financial security, even in uncertain financial times. We still want a loving marriage, even as the divorce rates soar. We still want peace in our time, even as the threat of nuclear holocaust continues. And when the realities of our lives are confronted by our unreal expectations, the result is problems. The immediacy of the world bombards us until we are immune, or seemingly immune, to what is going on. In actuality, we become very vulnerable.

TRAUMATIC TIMES

The headlines in newspapers today read like grade B movie plots: murder, mayhem, and fear unleashed on a helpless public. These are turbulent times, with problems that were inconceivable to our ancestors. From political assassinations to the anxiety over AIDS, we are asked to cope with seemingly impossible conditions. On the surface, we do adjust—heroically. Political candidates have countless bodyguards. We buy products with protective, sealed-up caps. We no longer have sex indiscriminately.

But there is an underlying anxiety in most of us today. There is the real fear that what has always happened to other people in other times and places can be and is happening to us. People we love are getting divorced, tightening their belts, and dying from AIDS. We can no longer trust our spouses or ourselves. Our jobs hinge on mergers and global events among people we don't know and nations we never heard of. Young adults no longer believe in marriage, and they take courses in college that look only at the bottom line. Like Robert after his heart attack, we are feeling out of control. The incidence of heart attacks and other stress-related diseases has risen. Depression, paranoia, and anxiety attacks have become more prevalent. The world is feeling the effects of aftershock.

STOP THE WORLD, I WANT TO GET OFF

We can't change the world overnight. But we can change the way we react to the traumatic events around us. We don't have to suffer from aftershock.

Unfortunately, the nature of aftershock can often make it extremely difficult to diagnose. It can strike weeks, months, or even years after a traumatic event, one from which we thought we had completely recovered. An event in the present—good or bad—can trigger aftershock in someone who had supposedly recovered from the effects of the earlier trauma. Even more confusing is the fact that aftershock affects people at different times in different ways. One person might feel jumpy and have difficulty sleeping. Another might escape by sleeping too much. We are all individuals, and the way we deal with trauma will be just as varied as our reasons for feeling happy or sad or angry.

THE SIGNPOSTS UP AHEAD

As far-reaching and unique as aftershock is, there are five main "red-flag" situations where its symptoms can crop up, often unexpectedly.

FOR BETTER OR FOR WORSE

When we think of trauma, we automatically think *bad:* death, divorce, or a catastrophic world event. But positive events, especially unexpected ones, can be just as frightening, and what makes them so insidious is the fact that it's more difficult to recognize the aftershock symptoms when they occur, since they follow a supposedly happy event.

WHAT DID I DO TO DESERVE THIS?

It isn't fair but it is reality. Even good, honest people can suffer from injustice. There are times in everyone's life when traumatic events occur, leaving aftershock in their wake: a divorce after fifteen years of marriage, cancer, a pink slip at work.

John had been happily married—or so he thought—to his childhood sweetheart for ten years. When she told him she was in love with someone else and wanted a divorce, John went into shock. For over five years, he refused to date or to go out and experience new things. His aftershock resulted in wasted years, years when he could have been productive, happy, and enjoying life.

THE FAMILY CIRCLE

A family doesn't have to be close knit to feel the effects of aftershock. If someone in your family has suffered from a trauma—illness or death or even something as seemingly predictable as retirement—the chances are good that you too might suffer from aftershock's effects.

Even entire families can feel the effects of aftershock. "We'd have been all right if there hadn't been any mess," says Beth Jarrett, the mother in the Academy Award-winning movie *Ordinary People*. The mess she's talking about is the death of her oldest son, which ultimately resulted in her surviving son's suicide attempt and the disintegration of her family.

SEEING IS BELIEVING

No man is an island. Aftershock can also occur to someone who only witnesses a trauma, one who has nothing to do with the event but who has the misfortune to have been in the wrong place at the wrong time.

On June 9, 1865, Charles Dickens was on a train that had an accident. His coach was fine, but several others fell off a bridge, resulting in ten deaths and forty-nine injuries. Later, though physically unharmed, he became weak, so weak that he couldn't write more than a few words at a time, and he couldn't travel by train for a long while afterward. He was suffering from aftershock.

THE LADY OF THE LAMP

Nurses, doctors, police officers, technicians, good Samaritans—none are immune from the effects of aftershock. People who take care of traumatized victims often find themselves in pain. For these people, career burnout is a fact of life and a very real problem in health care today.

The gallows humor the medics used in M*A*S*H was as much a defense against aftershock and the agonies of the Korean War as it was a way for them to remove themselves from the patients they were treating. To feel their pain would destroy them. They would be lost.

Despite these sobering scenarios, all is *not* lost. There is good news about trauma. No, things can't be altered. What is, is. We can't change what has happened, but we *can* change the way we feel. There is help. Personal growth and health can actually be fostered faster during a crisis than in normal everyday existence. All our feelings, energies, and thoughts are centered around the crisis. This intense focus provides the fuel to push through the pain and forge through our problems fast. The air is quickly cleared, and armed with understanding we can come out of our crises stronger and better off than we were before.

ARE YOU OR SOMEBODY YOU LOVE SUFFERING FROM AFTERSHOCK?

Whether or not you suffer from aftershock depends on how you've dealt with trauma in the past, how well you handle stress, how you were raised as a child, and when you seek help. Think about yourself over the past few years. Have you been feeling out of sorts? Do you have the feeling that life has been slipping by?

Below is a series of statements presented under three headings: your work life, the world at large, and your personal life. Some describe hypothetical situations, others describe emotions, and still others may describe situations that are very real to you at this point in time. Take a few moments to look them over. See if they apply to you and your world—the way you feel right now—and ask yourself how you might feel if they happened to you. They will give you food for thought as you evaluate your own potential for suffering from aftershock.

YOUR CAREER AND WORKPLACE

1. The stock market fall affected you personally.
2. You are snapping at people at work.
3. Rumors about a takeover are flying in your office.
4. A colleague at work has just received a promotion.
5. You are considering retirement.
6. Your boss has been fired, and you have been asked to take over the position.
7. You have been given a reprimand by higher-ups.
8. You have been laid off.
9. You haven't been satisfied with your job for a long time but haven't been able to make a move.
10. You are about to go on a job interview.
11. It's your first sales conference in the new position.
12. You are contemplating a different career.

THE WORLD AT LARGE

13. You can't read a newspaper without wanting to scream or cry.
14. Someone you know has recently been the victim of a violent crime.
15. A car accident occurred right in front of you, and your first impulse was to run.
16. A flight you almost took just crashed.
17. AIDS has you so scared that it's becoming a phobia.
18. You think people are talking about you.

19   You are afraid to stay home alone.

20   There has recently been a robbery in your neighborhood.

21   You are a war veteran.

YOUR PERSONAL WORLD

22   You have just received some good news, and it makes you nervous.

23   Someone you were close to has died within the past three months.

24   You have been waking up in the middle of the night.

25   You have a recurrent nightmare.

26   You are drinking and/or smoking more.

27   You start crying while watching a situation comedy on television.

28   Your pet has recently died.

29   Your divorce has been final for two years now, and you are still feeling angry at your ex-spouse.

30   A close friend has just moved away.

31   You grew up in an alcoholic home.

32   You just won the lottery.

33   You took the plunge and had plastic surgery.

34   Your marriage is on the rocky road lately, and you can't put your finger on what's wrong.

35   You've been gaining weight lately.

36   No one understands you.

37   You feel all alone.

38   You have received a late-night phone call that announced bad news.

39   Whenever you leave the house, you have the feeling that you have left the water running or that the burner is still set on high.

40   You have become uncomfortable in elevators or in crowds.

41   The smallest errand feels like an awesome chore.

42   You have stopped exercising, or you are exercising too much.

43 **Your relationships never seem to last more than a few months.**

44 **When things go wrong it always seems to be all your fault.**

These statements reflect some of the warning signs of aftershock. If you have answered yes to more than twenty-three of them, the chances are you or someone you love are in aftershock.

But you don't have to be in pain. You don't have to despair. Help is available. In the next few chapters we will be going over the different symptoms of trauma and aftershock—and what it all means.

We might live in difficult times, but they are also times of vast possibilities. Crisis and stress allow us to see what our needs are, what our vulnerabilities are, and what we *could* be if we made the forces that create aftershock, work for us instead. Though Charles Dickens wrote "It was the best of times, it was the worst of times" over one hundred years ago, those words still apply today. Welcome to what could be the beginning of the best of all times.

WHAT IS TRAUMA?

E VERYTHING IS RELATIVE. A MANAGER WHO CAN'T afford his mortgage loses patience when a colleague complains about the bad service aboard her recent flight to the Caribbean. A woman whose baby is sick can't be bothered with her friend's fear of growing old. A family worried about making ends meet is not going to be sympathetic to a neighbor's anxiety in finding good live-in help. "One man's heaven is another man's hell" is an age-old truth. Like these more mundane examples, traumatic events can be relative, too.

It is important to understand that trauma is not aftershock, rather trauma is the crisis (whether man-made or wrought by a natural disaster) that can *cause* aftershock.

A telling example of traumatic crisis is the case of a patient I treated a few years back, a man I will call William. William had everything to live for, including a prestigious new job, a happy marriage, and a bright future, until he and his wife were in a horrendous car accident.

He almost died. In a matter of moments his life was irrevocably changed. Here, with certain facts changed to protect his anonymity, are his words from our first session conducted with my colleague, Dr. Arvin Glicksman:

> **WILLIAM: Coming back late that evening at 11:00 I was driving a convertible and we were just in Bermuda shorts. . . . We had our dog in the back seat and the top was on because we were cool from our day. . . . My headlights picked up a whole group of raccoons crossing the highway, and I veered to the right. . . . I didn't want to kill anything, so I went to the right and this sheer granite cliff was facing us, so I veered to the left to make sure that we didn't climb the granite cliff and killed a number of the raccoons and the blood and guts went underneath the front wheels. . . . And we plummeted over a cliff. . . . We skidded off and thundered over a cliff into a gulley between the north and south lanes of the highway and the top of the car ripped open and we were not wearing seat belts and both my wife and I were found roughly about sixty feet from the car. . . .**

There is no doubt that this man was recounting a traumatic experience. It was sudden, it was shocking, and it changed his view of the world for good, as the following dialogue during that same session, shows:

> **QUESTION: Has the crisis changed your values in any way, your relationship to your wife, to colleagues, the family?**
> **WILLIAM: Yes, very much so. Both my wife and myself. My wife changed dramatically. . . . Since the accident . . . my wife came to the conclusion that no longer is she going to permit the world to insult her, under any circumstances. . . . Since the accident one might say now, "I don't give a damn. In other words, I'm going to do what I want to do."**

Fortunately, William and his wife recovered from their traumatic crisis; they have both become more assertive and more open with each other than before their highway crash.

Others are not as lucky. Thousands of men back from Vietnam are still feeling the effects of years spent slithering through the jungle; living with an eroding, constant fear; and fighting an unrecognizable foe. In the movie *Platoon*, Charlie Sheen, his innocence irrevocably lost, said of his leaders and his enemies, "They are both inside of me."

War, illness, horrendous accident—all are easy to identify as trauma. But some traumatic crisis are more subtle: a slowly eroding marriage, an alcoholic environment, a missed promotion. Even something as seemingly inconsequential as a fight with a friend or a flat tire on a country road can spell trauma for some. You might not see a promotion, a wedding, or any other positive event as traumatic, but these too have brought people to me, seeking relief from their fears and anxieties. For one woman, the walk down the aisle was a terrifying experience, even though she loved and wanted to be with the man she was to marry. Another woman who seemingly had everything—a family, a career, a lovely home—discovered she was miserable. She used a self-destructive affair to cure her boredom—temporarily.

The fact is that trauma wears many hats. And in any guise, it can have far-reaching effects long after the crisis has passed.

The Diagnostic and Statistical Manual of Mental Disorders (DSM-III), the bible for psychiatric diagnosis, defines trauma as "a psychologically traumatic event that is generally outside the range of usual human experience." But through my own experiences and those of my patients, I have found trauma and its resulting confusion to demand a much broader definition. A traumatic crisis is in actuality a turning point in the course of anything life offers—from good news to bad, from personal injury to upward mobility. After a trauma, things are not the same, nor will they ever be again.

Because traumatic events can cause such tremendous personal and worldwide upheavals, we must accept them—and understand them. Only then can we go on with our lives.

A TRAUMA IS A TRAUMA IS A TRAUMA

Without a basic understanding of color, an artist would be hard pressed to paint. Without a basic knowledge of bull and bear markets, a stockbroker would find it impossible to trade. Before you can recognize and treat a trauma's aftershock problem, you must first identify exactly what a trauma is.

There are six basic characteristics that make a trauma a trauma, regardless of the actual event. Some traumas exhibit all six characteristics; others as few as one. But they all signal a crisis and the possibility of aftershock later on. I will go over them one by one:

TO EVERYTHING THERE IS A SEASON—or the Element of Expected Versus Unexpected News

Joan's grandmother lived until a ripe old age. She was ninety-five when she fell on the ice and broke her pelvis. In the hospital, she contracted pneumonia and her body gave out. Joan mourned, but she knew she had been lucky to have her grandmother around as long as she did. Already in her thirties, Joan had married and given birth to a baby boy and had recently gone back to graduate school. All this her grandmother had seen and celebrated. Death is a traumatic experience for the survivors. But Joan's family *expected* the eventual death of the ninety-five-year-old grandmother. The family mourned her passing, tears were shed, but the death took place at an advanced age and in an acceptable way.

Ruth, on the other hand, died at 14, a victim of leukemia. She had been in and out of hospitals more days than she had been in school. Her parents knew everything about the disease; she herself had a knowledge of hospitals far beyond her years. Ruth had gone into remission twice, but these spells were hopelessly short lived. She was growing steadily weaker. Her death was inevitable, a mere matter of time. There was no surprise when Ruth breathed her last, but it was still *unexpected*. In the scheme of life, no one expects the death of a fourteen-year-old girl. Children should not have to die.

Though not fatal, Billy's accident was also unexpected. He had been planning a skiing trip to Colorado throughout his first semester in college. He had been skiing since he was a child and was a good, cautious skier, a natural athlete who took care of himself. Nobody could foresee that he would twist his ankle on a snow-covered branch and would fall on a nearby boulder, his leg broken in three places. Billy eventually recovered, but today in his mid-thirties he walks with a limp. And he has yet to get back on skis.

OUT OF THE BLUE—or the Element of Sudden Shock

No news is not necessarily good news. When a traumatic crisis comes out of the blue, without time for preparation, the results are sudden and total shock, a sometimes cruel and unusual punishment.

Take the case of Sean, a professor in his mid-forties, vibrant and alive. For years, he had played tennis three days a week during his lunch hour. Somehow he managed to help with his daughter's homework when he got home and always find time on the weekends for day trips with the entire family. When anyone talked about Sean, it was always with the highest praise—even after he dropped dead of a fatal heart attack one afternoon on the tennis court. There had been no signs, no symptoms of heart trouble or escalating blood pressure. Sean had seemed in the peak of health. His death was so unexpected and sudden that even he had not prepared sufficiently. It took years for his estate to be settled.

For Ellen, a former secretary, it was a positive trauma that took her by surprise. For five months, she had stopped religiously, twice a week, at her local drugstore to pick up a lottery ticket. She always wanted to win, but she knew the odds against her. Then one Saturday it really happened. Ellen won and became a millionaire overnight.

This is the stuff of dreams for countless players every week. But for Ellen it was a severe shock. She found her life turned upside down in a matter of days. She was no longer the Ellen her friends knew and loved. She became paranoid, unsure of which people were befriending her and why. Everyone, even her own family, had their hand out for more. Ellen quit her job; she bought some new clothes and changed her lifestyle. But she was floundering, suddenly unsure of who she was and where she belonged. She was no longer accepted by her old group of friends, nor did she fit into more conventional, upper-class circles. Eventually, she joined a lottery millionaires' self-help group and learned to cope with her new-found wealth with other winners.

Whether sudden shock or expected news, the intensity of an event is based on the third characteristic element of trauma, your past.

BACKWARD GLANCE—or the Element of Personal History

T.S. Eliot wrote that "all past time, present time, and future time is one time." Nowhere is this more true than when you are the victim of a traumatic crisis. If you have been through a divorce, you will be worried that it will happen again, even if your second marriage is a good one. If you have ever been burglarized, the chances are you will overreact to a sound heard late at night. Similarly, if one of your parents died at an early age when you were still a child, the death of your pet dog or cat would probably affect you more than someone who had never known loss.

I first saw Margaret as a patient after her business failed. One day she had suddenly found herself crying over the steering wheel of her car, convinced she was "the bad child that nobody could love." Was Margaret simply overreacting to a common enough trauma—the loss of her business? No, not if you understand her past. As a child, her parents had taught her to keep her emotions in check, to show a mask of strength to the world. Margaret had learned her lessons too well.

As a young adult she nursed her parents as they battled against consecutive terminal illnesses; she did not allow herself to cry at their funerals. She inherited the family business and plunged herself wholeheartedly into it, deriving self-esteem and satisfaction in doing her job well. When the firm declared bankruptcy, she had nothing to fall back on; the grief she had held in all those years finally came out.

In Margaret's case, the trauma of her failing business triggered the traumas from her childhood, intensifying the crisis.

Jim, too, brought his unresolved past to the present. When he said, "I do," he was vowing to make his marriage work. Not only did he love Kathy with all his heart, but he remembered the pain he had experienced as a child when his parents divorced. "I have to make this marriage work," he would say over beers with his friends. "I'm not going to make the same mistakes my parents did." Unfortunately, Jim and Kathy grew apart, and she finally filed for divorce. The trauma hit Jim much harder than it would have had he not come from a broken home.

FOUL PLAY—or the Element of Unfairness

History has always had its irony, its lack of fair play in meting out justice. Henry VIII killed two of his wives on a whim. The children of the Czar were murdered because they had the misfortune of a royal last name. The Indians sold New York Island for a song and were kicked out for their trouble. And millions were led to the slaughter because they were Jews.

Nowhere it seems, is the sense of injustice more encompassing than in today's world. From the threat of nuclear holocaust to AIDS, unfairness looms over the eighties like a low-flying plane. Thus:

It's not fair that a young man dies of AIDS from his first and only sexual encounter.

It's not fair that we must live in a world where hijacking innocent people on a plane is a way of life.

It's not fair that a husband divorces his wife after she has supported him throughout his years of medical school.

It's not fair that a young girl dies after being sexually or otherwise brutally abused.

It's not fair that a woman who has been healthy all her life develops breast cancer.

It's not fair that you receive a promotion only to find that people envy your success.

It's not fair that you have studied long and hard in law school, only to find that there is no job to be had.

The list goes on. We can be mad as hell and refuse to take anymore, but that won't stop a traumatic event from taking place. Trauma and its unfair aspect is the stuff of novels, plays, poems—and life.

THE FICKLE FINGER OF FATE—or the Element of Control

A feeling of powerlessness goes hand in hand with a sense of unfairness. There was no way to stop Mt. St. Helens from spewing volcanic ash onto the outlying communities. When Martin Luther King was assassinated, there was no way to bring him back to life. On a more personal level, there is nothing more frustrating than watching others decide your fate.

When Shearson Lehman Brothers, Inc. bought E.F. Hutton before Christmas 1987, the 18,000 Hutton people were feeling the traumatic effects. A senior analyst reported in *USA Today* "There have been crying sessions in people's offices for the past week and a half. It's like living in occupied France." The president of Hutton had even been hospitalized for a stress-related illness. Unfair, yes. And more than anything else, productive of a complete feeling of helplessness. Eighteen thousand people and not one of them could stop the merger, not one of them could change the strategies planned, presumably for months, behind anonymous conference room doors.

POINTING THE FINGER—or the Element of Blame

Michael always considered himself a careful driver. He had been driving for thirty years without even a parking ticket to his credit. He had driven in blizzards, in fog, and on back-country roads. People liked to drive with Michael; he inspired confidence.

Michael also liked to drink, especially at parties. Since everyone else was sipping cocktails, no one particularly noticed the way he was guzzling the vodka and tonics at his best friend's annual New Year's Eve bash. Even if they did, people wouldn't be concerned. After all, Michael knew how to handle liquor, just like he knew how to handle a car.

It was three o'clock when Michael rose unsteadily to his feet, ready to leave. When his friend expressed concern, suggesting that Michael stay the night, he told him not to worry. "Get me behind the wheel with a cup of coffee and I'm instantly sober," he declared. Drunken drivers hang out all night in bars; they are irresponsible people. Not Michael. At 3:17 that same morning, Michael hit an oncoming car, killing a teenage couple instantly. Michael was shocked: "It couldn't have happened to me!" But it did. And he had no one to blame for the trauma but himself.

A woman blames herself for a broken-up marriage. A man considers it his fault that he has been laid off. A child fears it was her temper tantrum that caused her father's death.

Blame translates into guilt, and intensifies aftershock. No matter who points the finger, and at whom, blame is a crucial element of aftershock.

Take a moment to look at the chart below. It shows the different elements that make up several sample traumas, illustrating the fact that a life-changing crisis does not have to be a devastating event, like a violent crime or a war experience, to be deemed traumatic and capable of causing aftershock. In this chart I do not wish to imply that being fired from your job is the same as fighting in a war, or surviving a natural disaster. Clearly, these experiences are worlds apart. But I do wish to point out that there can be common elements to a variety of experiences, that help explain why even the birth of a child might cause aftershock.

	Expected or Unexpected	Sudden	Past Hist.	Unfair	Control	Blame
Death of Spouse	✓	✓	✓	✓	✓	✓
War	✓	✓	✓	✓	✓	✓
Murder	✓	✓		✓	✓	✓
Job Loss	✓	✓	✓	✓	✓	✓
Divorce	✓	✓	✓	✓	✓	✓
Natural Disaster	✓	✓		✓	✓	
Miscarriage	✓		✓	✓	✓	✓
Promotion	✓	✓	✓		✓	
Marriage	✓		✓			
Birth	✓		✓		✓	

Time heals most wounds. When the dust finally settles, the trauma might seem a distant memory. But aftershock has yet to make an appearance. It occurs after the traumatic event, and its symptoms can make it look like an entirely unrelated condition. But one thing is certain: aftershock can hurt if it isn't recognized and treated. In the next chapter, I will examine the repercussions of trauma to help you discover exactly what aftershock is and why it occurs.

WHAT IS AFTERSHOCK?

$$3$$

IN HIS EXCELLENT BOOK, *Posttraumatic Stress Disorder: Diagnosis, Treatment, and Legal Issues* (Praeger, 1984), Dr. C. B. Scrignar describes an unusual case:

From Monday to Friday, Rosemarie's morning routine never varied. She would get off the bus near her office, stop at the coffee shop on the corner, and order her regular takeout coffee and bran muffin. She would enter her building, buy a paper from the newsstand, and take the elevator up to her office. Before the day's work began, she would eat her muffin and drink her coffee as she skimmed the news. By 9:00, she would be returning early morning calls.

This particular Tuesday was different. Rosemarie was at her desk, eating her muffin and sipping her coffee as she read the newspaper. She glanced down for a moment at her muffin and discovered a dead cockroach in the uneaten piece. Rosemarie gagged. She ran to the rest room and threw up her breakfast. She was sweating and she had the shakes. Unable to work, she left the office and went home. The coffee shop offered a profuse apology and reimbursement. But Rosemarie was not interested in any monetary gain; her focus was already beyond lawsuits and retribution.

She became obsessive about disease and cockroaches. She was certain that the cold she had developed was due to the half-cooked bug. She had her apartment exterminated an inordinate number of times, twice each week under a standing arrangement. She became compulsively clean, refusing to eat in coffee shops and restaurants. She had recurring nightmares about crawling bugs.

Six months after the incident, Rosemarie couldn't bring herself to go to the office. She couldn't work and she lost her job. What might have been a repulsive but ultimately insignificant event for someone else had become a highly traumatic life-changing crisis for Rosemarie. She had become a victim of severe aftershock.

REACTION TIME

Rosemarie's Kafkaesque experience contained several of the elements of trauma, outlined in the previous chapter, that contribute to aftershock. It was sudden, it was unexpected, it was out of her control, and it changed her life. But at first there were no intimations of aftershock. Rosemarie's initial reaction was perfectly normal. Anyone finding a cockroach in a half-eaten muffin would be totally repulsed. Vomiting and nausea would be considered an appropriate reaction, as would a call to the exterminator and an initial avoidance of coffee shops and muffins.

Similarly, it makes sense that if you were involved in a car accident, you would be wary the next few times you got behind the wheel, or if you had just survived a major flood, the next few drops of rain would make you shudder. In fact, a highly-charged reaction to a shocking event is vital to your emotional and physical health. It is only when that reaction takes over your life that there are problems. And, more times than not, the responses you have to the traumatic events in your life *are* healthy, even though they might not seem so at the time. Here is proof.

THE PRIMAL SCREAM

When a child falls and scrapes a knee, it will immediately start to cry. Mommy! is a familiar refrain for parents everywhere, causing more overflowing sinks and more burned dinners than any other exclamation. It's a cry that follows straight through to adulthood. When faced with a life or death situation, men at war have called out for their mothers. *Mutter! Mater! Ma! Mere! Emau!* Mom!—their outcry is heard through the ages.

This shout for help, for release, usually occurs during or right after a stressful life event. Why? As Dr. Mardi Horowitz states in an article published in *Hospital and Community Psychiatry*, "The immediate response to a serious life event is often alarm, accompanied by strong emotion, most often fear. This initial appraisal leading to a short period of outcry occurs as one processes the crude implications of the event . . . an alarm reaction that interrupts ordinary activities and expresses warning signals." Something frightens us, we stop everything and cry out for comfort, aware only of our fear. Perfectly natural.

But sometimes this outcry stage occurs later, when the experience of the trauma has a chance to sink in. How many people have heard the news of a parent's death only to cry about it days or even months later when their minds finally accept the fact.

When your coping efforts are no longer necessary, when you are alone and your defenses are down, you will, either vocally or silently, cry out with tears of sadness.

SORRY, WRONG NUMBER

Normal reactions to a shocking event also include some denial. When you cannot take the shock of a stressful life event, you will deny it, modulating your emotional responses into tolerable, time-spaced doses. You will go to the office and pretend to conduct business as usual. You will do a laundry and clean house if you have just gotten divorced.

Think of it: If you dissolved a medication filled with time-release capsules and swallowed its entire contents, it could be lethal. The timed release of the ingredients prevents too much dosage and assures a supply of just enough medicine to keep you going. So too with shock. Small amounts of reality build up resilience and adaptability to the trauma. If you integrated the entire shocking event into your system all at once, you could go mad.

WE INTERRUPT THIS PROGRAM . . .

When you suffer a shock, denial is often accompanied by an intrusive stage—a time when emotions flood in, when the traumatic event appears fresh in your mind. These emotions are usually triggered by a haunting smell or sound or a flash of something familiar caught in the corner of your eye. You might find yourself weeping at the slightest cue: a TV situation comedy, a song on the radio, a surly salesperson in the corner store. You might find yourself acting compulsively, driven to finish that spring-cleaning job or that closet that needs organizing, or rigidly keeping to a schedule that has room for flexibility.

These inner sensations and feelings can be intense, so intense that they may actually conjure up visual images and "spirits." A grief-stricken mourner might actually "feel" or "sense" his dead loved one sitting at the table or in the easy chair by the fire. Though a powerful notion and the stuff of great fiction, these paranormal experiences are more likely the intense emotional feelings conjured up during this intrusive stage. Called *hypnogogic* phenomena when they occur right before sleep and *hypnopompic* phenomena when they occur just before awakening, these so-called paranormal hallucinations are the visual, sensory perceptions that easily float into your uncluttered, half-conscious mind.

This unpredictable, startling quality of the intrusive stage scares people into believing they are going crazy. Wrong: This stage is a part of the normal reaction to a stressful life event, especially to one who has gone through a denial phase and in whose brain the reaction has been lying dormant. Healing is a process and it takes time. Like building a house from the ground up, it must be done in stages.

THE SIX STAGES OF EMOTION

Psychiatrist Elisabeth Kübler-Ross in her landmark book, *On Death and Dying* (Macmillan, 1969) outlined six stages of acceptance when a patient learns he or she is suffering from a terminal illness. These same six stages of emotion can apply to anyone who has suffered or is suffering from a traumatic stressful life event.

[1]   **Denial.** When faced with a negative life-changing event like the death of a loved one or a prowler on the loose, the first reaction is "This isn't happening to me!" Similar responses occur in people who have just experienced a change for the better, such as getting that promotion or winning a lottery. Their "I don't believe it!" can be heard throughout the room.

[2]   **Anger.** After denial comes anger—at yourself, at your family and friends, at the world at large. "Why did this happen to me!" "It's not fair!" "I hate you!"

[3]   **Bargaining.** Bargaining or negotiating is third: "Please God, if only I get out of this alive, I'll be a good person from now on. I promise."

[4]   **Depression.** How many of us have suffered from a gray view of the world after a loss—be it a job, a marriage, or a death? Freud, back in the earlier part of the century, found depression to be the normal reaction to grief, with a characteristic lack of interest in sex, in outside activities, and in oneself.

[5]   **Acceptance.** Finally, as we work through the depression stage, we begin to accept what has happened. The crisis becomes integrated within our mind, as is the realization that what is—is—and can't be changed.

[6]   **Hope.** This new view of the world brings with it hope and the chance for a brighter future.

If you are a healthy person who experiences a trauma, you will go through each of these six stages in sequence. Problems arise when you get stuck in any one of these stages, or when you miss one. A newly divorced woman who can't get angry at her ex-spouse has not completed the healing cycle. A man who continues to be depressed after losing his job will never get to accept what has happened nor will he find hope for his future. Both situations are fertile ground for aftershock.

HIGH ANXIETY

Obviously if you had a choice, you would pick winning a lottery ticket over contracting breast cancer or eating a wormy apple over having to shoot to kill. But you can't choose your traumatic events any more than you can choose your parents or your height. And even if you could pick and choose your life events, there would still be no guarantee that your reactions would be as you expect.

It's almost impossible to gauge how you will react to a life event. Rosemarie's reaction to finding a bug in her muffin was as severe as that of a woman who was a victim of rape. The fact is that the severity of a traumatic event has no bearing on the severity of our response. As we have seen, a person can suffer aftershock from a positive trauma, a negative trauma, or even one that is relatively minor.

Plato defined reality as one's perception of it. He could have been talking about trauma and its aftershock. If you are extremely anxious before, during, or after a stressful life event, the chances are you will perceive it as highly traumatic and increase your chances of getting aftershock. In his book, *Posttraumatic Stress Disorder*, Dr. C. B. Scrignar outlines five levels of anxiety that have a direct bearing on whether or not you will suffer from a trauma's aftermath.

⚡ Level 5: panic—The danger zone of doom and gloom, complete with sudden panic attacks and terrifying thoughts of going crazy

⚡ Level 4: severe—Trembling or shaking, fainting, hot flashes, and other physical reactions

⚡ Level 3: moderate—Moderate anxiety coupled with stomach aches or trouble breathing

⚡ Level 2: mild—Mild symptoms like edginess, tenseness, or nervousness

⚡ Level 1: normal—No anxiety, calm

Even if you see yourself at level four or five, you can ease your feelings of hopelessness and anxiety over time. Time does heal and soothe. But if you remain at a high level of stress, if you have been stuck in any one of the six emotional stages of the acceptance process, or if your denial and destructive periods become more and more intense, you may be suffering from aftershock and denying yourself a full and happy life.

THE STRAW THAT BROKE
THE CAMEL'S BACK

It's an old expression, but it's applicable to trauma. You can cope and cope with a trauma—until you can't. You can sweep your feelings under the rug for just so long, before aftershock demands the floor. The trauma might be long gone, but your ordeal is not over. Even if your accurate recollections of an event abate, you can be left with its residue, free-floating anxiety, panic attacks, and paralyzing fear.

How does aftershock begin and how does it work its insidious spell? Here are several theories based on research done by specialists in posttraumatic stress disorder, that can be applied to aftershock.

THE "ALLERGIC" REACTION

The first time Eleanore was given penicillin for a bronchitis attack, she developed a minor rash. Though it disappeared after she stopped the medication, no correlation was made between the penicillin and the rash. Eleanore completely discounted it; everyone breaks out occasionally. Unfortunately, she had another attack a year later, and her doctor, not knowing about the rash, once again prescribed penicillin. This time Eleanore's reaction was much more severe. After taking only one pill she could barely walk; she had chills. Her doctor immediately recognized Eleanore's penicillin allergy. She told Eleanore that if she took just one more pill, she could very well go into convulsions and die.

Eleanore's story is a common pattern in many allergic reactions. The first time one takes the medication, the reaction is subtle even after a large dose. The second time around, there is a much stronger reaction, after only a minimal amount of exposure.

This same "allergic" reaction can apply to aftershock. Witness this story of a man based upon a report by K. Garb and colleagues in the *British Journal of Psychiatry* who fought in the Israeli army: Diagnosed as having aftershock after a friend died in his arms during Israel's 1973 Yom Kippur War, Rubin eventually recovered. Nine years later, he had successfully raised a family, managed a business, and was living a seemingly contented life. When Rubin was called up again for the Lebanon war of 1982, he suffered a tremendous anxiety attack, and he actually collapsed when he came to his unit. Just like Eleanore's severe anaphylactic attack after taking just one penicillin tablet, Rubin's severe aftershock reaction occurred after only a minimal exposure to trauma.

Another case reported by Garb and colleagues in the *British Journal of Psychiatry* is that of Rita, a woman who as a child survived the Holocaust. She recovered and learned to accept the deaths of her family in the camps. Yet although it was not in her conscious mind, Rita still remembered the cry of a young girl, her shouts of "Mama!" as she was pushed into a "delousing" line. When Rita gave birth to her first child, she went into a severe depression, remembering that lost child from years before.

THE AVALANCHE PRINCIPLE

Another form of PTSD can be called an avalanche effect. Just as an avalanche starts with a few pebbles that, gathering momentum, turn into a landslide, so too can stress turn into traumatic aftershock.

If you are facing a traumatic, stressful life event that does not ease, such as money pressures that keep snowballing or a sinking, eroding marriage, your stress level will go higher and higher and your reaction will become more and more debilitating. Here, aftershock is slower growing, but its effects can be as deadly as an unexpected, sudden crash.

NETWORKING

Think of a networking colleague at a cocktail party, tracing a path through a crowded room of potential clients. Then think of a traumatic event, indelibly etched onto the human brain via the various chemicals in the brain acting as the "acid" that etches the event "in stone" in the brain's passageways. (Studies have shown these "acids" to be vasopressins and ACTH, two of the chemicals that are released by the brains of laboratory animals undergoing stress.)

Some experts theorize that these newly-etched passageways might lay dormant for a while until a stimulus in the present brings back the past, a reaction symptomatic of posttraumatic stress disorder. Here is an example based upon a case reported by Dr. Roger Pitman. A Korean vet in his late fifties was sitting at the kitchen table, reading a paper and drinking coffee while the TV set was on. The news was being reported and the sound of a helicopter was heard. Suddenly the man became dazed, complained of nausea, and shouted, "They're bringing in more!" He then collapsed into a deep sleep. When he woke up, he was perfectly fine.

What happened here is that the helicopter noise stimulated those etched passageways in his brain, bringing the past brilliantly alive. If he had been watching television instead of merely listening, he would have seen visual proof that he was in the present. But with only the sound going, he went back in time. The vet said later that if he had actually seen the helicopter on TV, he would have stayed firmly rooted in reality.

THE THREE Es

Another theory, developed by Dr. C. B. Scrignar, centers on the three Es: environment, encephalic (thought) events, and endogenous (physical) events. All three work together in a spiraling effect to cause aftershock symptoms. Let's go over each of them, one by one.

Environment

Whether sudden, unfair, or unexpected, one thing is certain: an event is a trauma if it has an impact on you. If an event gives you stress, if it changes your life in some way, or if it acts upon any of your five senses, there is no doubt you are experiencing a traumatic life event. And the chances are you will feel a certain amount of anxiety and find yourself in the throes of aftershock.

Encephalic Events

These are your thoughts, your fantasies, and your beliefs—all that you dream and think after a traumatic event. After you have experienced a stressful life event, it is recorded in your brain, ready to play back like a cassette in a VCR. When the "tape" plays back over and over again seemingly without your control, the trauma will continue to stay fresh in your mind, retraumatizing you to the event. Every time Rosemarie bit into food, her video cassette played back in her mind, complete with a recording that suggested how she could have eaten the cockroach in her muffin, how it could have been alive, and other macabre scenarios.

Colleagues and friends might perceive a person suffering from a posttraumatic shock as moody, obsessive, self-indulgent, and unwilling to put the past to rest. But in actuality, it is the continuous tape, rather than the will of the sufferer that is keeping the trauma very much alive and real. The person is completely sensitized to the event and to any stimulus that might set it off. Unfortunately this heightened awareness and anxiety can spread to other areas and cause financial conflicts, work problems, sexual dysfunction, and more. Though these problems might look like isolated concerns, they are really offshoots from the one traumatic event. They are very real affects of aftershock.

Endogenous Events

These are the physical sensations that add more fuel to anxiety's fire. The stress resulting from the trauma sets off the autonomic nervous system, which in turn creates such physical symptoms as trembling, migraines, stomach aches, and panic attacks. These symptoms are so real and so fraught with anxiety that victims are convinced they are sick even when they have gotten a clean bill of health from their doctors. They will go from specialist to specialist, their world so filled with their physical ailments that the trauma that started it all is forgotten.

Environment, encephalic events, endogenous events—these three elements are intimately connected in a spiraling effect, keeping aftershock alive after the stressful life event has passed.

Here is how it works. *Environment* sets the stimuli in motion—the "on" switch on the VCR that keeps the *encephalic* cassette tape running in your brain. This running tape, in turn, keeps the anxiety going strong and creates the anxiety-producing *endogenous* physical ailments. These physical health worries become a main focus and heighten a person's awareness of *environment* stimuli. If the initial traumatic event is stressful enough to reach his or her threshold, no person—no matter how strong, stable, or normal—can be immune from aftershock.

FIGHT OR FLIGHT

Almost everyone has heard of the "fight or flight" phenomenon, the reaction that sends a rush of adrenaline into your system when you are confronted with danger. When confronted by a threat or by a situation that we perceive as a threat, our nervous and glandular systems become activated, resulting in the faster heartbeat, muscular contraction, and more rapid breathing that prepares one for fight—or flight if we think our enemy too strong. The change in physiology caused by the fight or flight response puts stress on the body, and if the emergency situation does not dissipate soon, this added stress will become a health hazard.

For primitive man, this adrenaline rush meant daily survival. Without its stimulus a Neanderthal man, in the path of an angry leopard or a rabid wild boar, would never have had a chance.

But today in most situations, that surge of adrenaline has nowhere to go. When you are confronted with a stressful, traumatic event, that rush of adrenaline becomes an uninvited guest. You can't very well pummel the boss that has just screamed at you nor can you smash the Wall Street trading floor when you have just lost a bundle. Instead, you have an anxious feeling that has no outlet, a jumpiness that needs release.

These theories of aftershock are only a part of the story. The rest, as they say, is history.

THE HISTORY OF AFTERSHOCK AND ITS BATTLE SCARS

As long as there is life to live, there will be traumatic ups and downs. And humankind will continue ad infinitum to react—sometimes with courage, sometimes with joy, and sometimes with fear.

In the primitive world, men and women were terrified by lightning and other natural phenomena. They would lay on the war paint and the superstitious baubles to keep the angry gods at bay. Nightmares became prophecy, and fear became the frenzied ritual of sacrifice. Traumatized men who refused to hunt or kill would presumably be killed themselves.

As early as 1700 B.C., in Hammurabi's Babylonian army, revenge was considered a just reaction to traumatic experience in battle. Ancient Greek and Roman writers created epic poetry about the traumas of men in war. Who can say for sure that Cleopatra's suicide was not an aftershock reaction brought on by the traumas of losing the man and the empire she loved?

But these thoughts aside, the first aftershock research was an outcome of war. It was here, on the battlefields, that physicians treated men in combat firsthand. And it was here too that physicians first saw signs of psychological ailments they termed battle fatigue and shell shock. As far back as 1871, Dr. Jacob Mendes DaCosta discovered an erratic heartbeat in some young Civil War veterans, with no apparent physical cause. He dubbed this phenomenon "irritable heart," and later any posttraumatic symptom was labeled DaCosta's syndrome.

During the Russo-Japanese War of 1904–1905, men were officially treated for psychological disturbances on the front line. And, in 1919, Sir Thomas Lewis discovered unaccountable nausea, anxiety attacks, fatigue, and chest pains in World War I soldiers. Da Costa's syndrome was changed to his "soldier's heart" and the "Effort Syndrome."

America was one of the last countries to recognize the psychological nature of combat stress. In 1943, only 18 percent of the Fifth Army soldiers suffering from battle fatigue were able to go back to the front lines in Italy. One year later, psychiatrists were assigned to the infantry division, and the figure rose to 85 percent!

Ironically, America caught up with the rest of the world with the Vietnam War, the war that finally brought PTSD to the forefront. A staggering number of the 3.5 million men who served there were—and are—affected by aftershock, in some cases twenty years after the fact.

WHAT THE HELL ARE WE FIGHTING FOR?

On April 26, 1979, the Senate Veterans Affairs Committee filed a formal report to authorize the Veterans Administration to recognize and treat PTSD among Vietnam vets. Why it took so long for the government to act is not clear. Perhaps it was because the whole country wanted to forget the war. Perhaps our governmental officials did not want to think there was anything different about Vietnam; perhaps they believed that the same benefits given their fathers and grandfathers should apply to the Vietnam vets. And some officials may have viewed the bill's supporters as former Vietnam-War protestors, who had not supported our country during the years of fighting.

When the bill was finally authorized, only $9 million out of a total V.A. budget of $23 billion was allowed—and for only two years. But by 1981, the need for PTSD treatment became undeniable, with between 500,000 and 800,000 PTSD-diagnosed vets. A veto from President Reagan was overruled, and the bill received a new three-year extension with a hefty budget of $31 million.

Why was this war different? Why did it cause so much after-shock? For many reasons. First of all, the Vietnam War contained all the elements of trauma inherent in any war:

⟩ The maiming and the killing that has suddenly become so-cially acceptable

⟩ The awareness that war is an entirely man-made disaster

⟩ The inversion of value systems

But the Vietnam War also had elements that no other war has had. Here were young boys being shucked away from their peacetime homes to be relocated and de-individualized in the steamy, alien jungles of Southeast Asia. Here, for at least a year, they were surrounded by daily death and devastation. Here they were wasted by snipers and "friendly fire." Here they found a daily diet of terror—as well as readily available drugs that lowered their strength and their resistance to taking orders.

Add to this stressful, nightmarish environment the fact that within hours the soldiers were whisked back to America, where they received no support, no homecoming, and, for 600,000 to 1,000,000 vets, a less-than-honorable discharge and unemployment. Whatever guilt they suf-fered from combat was combined with an overwhelming rage at those who had stayed at home.

For many of these vets, a psychotic reality of war and daily mas-sacre could not blend in with the peacetime reality of America. They developed symptoms of paranoia; they still expected to die. As a Viet-nam medic, waiting in an ambush, once said, "I had to permit my old reality to slide away through a membrane."

This seemingly new problem needed a new psychiatric classifica-tion. PTSD became a full-fledged official disease and by law covered by medical insurance.

DSM ZONE

The Diagnostic and Statistical Manual of Mental Disorders, Third Edi-tion, Revised, (DSM-III-R) is more than a psychiatrist's tool. Published in 1980 and revised in 1986–1987, it assigns diagnostic codes to each disorder. These codes, in turn, are used by health insurance companies to reimburse patients. Consequently, mental health professionals will use the *DSM-III* to fill out the forms they must submit—but the result is not so much an accurate appraisal as a bureaucratic attempt to make a neat and tidy pigeon hole, to create a black-and-white situation out of something that is much more complicated. It's similar to the partners in a dissolving marriage trying to explain what happened totally in terms of dollars and cents.

But being categorized in *DSM-III-R* does give a disorder a credibility it might not otherwise have. Thanks to the Vietnam War, post-traumatic stress disorder is now listed under the general category of anxiety disorder. It now has a significance in the psychiatric community and in the world at large. But because its definition is narrowly confined to the horrific traumas of war, *DSM-III-R* discounts many of the traumas I have already talked about, as well as the ones I will be outlining in the next section. However, the manual is useful as a jumping-off point for further study.

Here then, before we go any further, is a partial listing of the *DSM-III-R* qualifications for PTSD. (The entire listing can be found in the appendix.)

A   The person has experienced an event that is outside the range of usual human experience and that would be markedly distressing to almost anyone, e.g., serious threat to one's life or physical integrity; serious threat or harm to one's children, spouse, or other close relatives and friends; sudden destruction of one's home or community; or seeing another person who has recently been, or is being, seriously injured or killed as the result of an accident or physical violence.

B   The traumatic event is persistently reexperienced in at least one of the following ways:
  1   recurrent and intrusive distressing recollections of the event (in young children, repetitive play in which themes or aspects of the trauma are expressed)
  2   recurrent distressing dreams of the event
  3   sudden acting or feeling as if the traumatic event were recurring (includes a sense of reliving the experience, illusions, hallucinations, and dissociative [flashback] episodes, even those that occur upon awakening or when intoxicated)

    4   intense psychological distress at exposure to events that symbolize or resemble an aspect of the traumatic event, including anniversaries of the trauma

C   Persistent avoidance of stimuli associated with the trauma or numbing of general responsiveness (not present before the trauma), as indicated by at least three of the following:

    1   efforts to avoid thoughts or feelings associated with the trauma

    2   efforts to avoid activities or situations that arouse recollections of the trauma

    3   inability to recall an important aspect of the trauma (psychogenic amnesia)

    4   markedly diminished interest in significant activities (in young children, loss of recently acquired developmental skills such as toilet training or language skills)

    5   feeling of detachment or estrangement from others

    6   restricted range of affect, e.g., unable to have loving feelings

    7   sense of a foreshortened future, e.g., does not expect to have a career, marriage, or children, or a long life

D   Persistent symptoms of increased arousal (not present before the trauma), as indicated by at least two of the following:

    1   difficulty falling or staying asleep

    2   irritability or outbursts of anger

    3   difficulty concentrating

    4   hypervigilance

    5   exaggerated startle response

    6   physiologic reactivity upon exposure to events that symbolize or resemble an aspect of the traumatic event (e.g., a woman who was raped in an elevator breaks out in a sweat when entering any elevator)

E   Duration of the disturbance (symptoms in B, C, and D) of at least one month.

Specify *delayed onset* if the onset of symptoms was at least six months after the trauma.*

---

* Source: American Psychiatric Association, Diagnostic and Statistical Manual of Mental Disorders, Third Edition, Revised. Washington, DC, American Psychiatric Association, 1987.

The key words in this list are "an event that is outside the range of usual human experience and that would be markedly distressing to almost anyone. . . ." We have already gone over the elements of trauma and have learned that any event, positive or negative, can be deemed a trauma. Though PTSD became a recognized clinical entity because of the Vietnam War, I believe its repercussions are much broader than its *DSM-III-R* definition implies. *And it is this broader definition that I have termed aftershock.* Yes, it is a reaction to war. Yes, it is a reaction to a violent crime. Yes, it is a reaction to a natural disaster. But aftershock is also much more than that.

MORE THAN ITS NAME

Depression has been around since the days of Ancient Egypt. Schizophrenia and anxiety were kept under lock and key in many a Victorian family's attic. But PTSD is a fairly new entry into our psychological vocabulary. Why? First of all, it's difficult to pinpoint its cause and effect. Symptoms don't crop up until a traumatic event has passed, sometimes years later. And the symptoms themselves are so common that they can fit many other disorders. Secondly, PTSD was only seen and studied in men in combat. In reality, more women suffer from aftershock than men—in a three-to-two ratio.

In fact, one study reports that 60 percent of all persons with symptoms of mental disorder had suffered from a traumatic life event two weeks before they showed any sign of illness. Only 20 percent of the people who suffered from a trauma *did not* have an aftershock reaction. And another study found that in the months following a traumatic life event, there is sixfold greater risk of suicide, a twofold greater risk of depression, and a slightly greater possibility of becoming schizophrenic—than in the period prior to the event.

And nowhere is aftershock more insidious than in children and in families. Let's see why this is so.

THE CHILDREN'S HOUR

"Childhood has no forebodings; But then, it is soothed by no memories of outlived sorrow."

(Author unknown)

The *DSM-III-R* classification cites the fact that PTSD can occur at any age, even childhood. But what it doesn't say is that children are *especially* vulnerable to a posttraumatic reaction to shock.

Like their growing bones and bodies, the brains of young children are not as well developed as in adults—especially the hippocampus, the part of the brain that controls and stores events in a specific time and place. The one part of the brain that *is* well developed, however, is the section that remembers feelings and sounds, an area that can trigger PTSD hallucinations in adults.

Problems arise when children experience a stressful life event. One of the key elements in preventing an aftershock reaction is the ability to place a traumatic event in its rightful time and place. Since children cannot neurologically and physically do that, they are forced to deal with the trauma using only the part of their brain that is developed, the hallucinatory area of memories and feelings.

Further, trauma affects children differently than it does adults. For example, divorce might be acceptable to two consenting adults—especially in today's world—but to their eight-year-old child, divorce can be a shocking event.

A FAMILY AFFAIR

In Anna Karenina, Leo Tolstoy wrote that "all happy families are like one another; each unhappy family is unhappy in its own way." When a member of the family is stricken with aftershock, it becomes everyone's problem. No one is immune to a father's layoff, to the birth of a new baby, or to a move to another city. Similarly, a teenager's bout with depression is going to affect the entire atmosphere of the house.

What makes this family connection even more vital is the fact that an aftershock victim desperately needs the support of family and friends. Without their understanding, they could actually hinder the victim's journey back to health.

Aftershock behavior can be passed down from one generation to another. Witness the story of Joan, whose mother began to abuse her physically. When Joan failed to make her bed one morning, her mother took out a belt and smacked her. It was only the beginning. Whenever Joan did something "bad," like ignoring her homework or forgetting to take out the garbage, she would get the belt. These stressful events completely traumatized the girl. She vowed that she would never act like her mother, that when she was a mother herself, she would only use understanding and kind words.

At first, Joan seemed to keep her promise. She raised a lovely daughter who had grown into a typical teen. Joan tried to reason with her daughter when she stayed on the phone all hours, when she refused to clean her room. But everything flew out the window the night Joan's daughter yelled at her. It was only teenage rebellion, but to Joan it was the last straw. Without thinking, she reached for the only role model life had offered her. She reached for the belt.

EMOTIONAL OUTLET

Emote means to act, and emotions are our way of acting out our reactions to trauma. Whatever the cause, whatever the event, there are five aftershock emotions that are universal. Delineated by Dr. M. J. Horowitz, Dr. George Mendelson, and others, they are

Fear
/ Of the trauma repeating. If someone you loved died, it can happen again to another person you love.
/ Of the victim's similarity to you. If someone you know has been a victim of a crime, you can be too.
/ Of aggressive loss of control. Anger can be a very scary thing, especially when you feel an inability to control yourself.
Worry
/ Over the failure to prevent the trauma. You couldn't stop the car crash and you are feeling ashamed and useless.
Rage
/ At anyone felt responsible. Everyone likes to blame someone, even if it's totally irrational.

⚡ At anyone lucky enough not to be involved. It's not fair that you are going bankrupt and the fortunes of all your friends are on the upswing.

Guilt

⚡ Over feeling such rage. In your heart of hearts, you know it isn't completely your husband's fault that you have been growing apart.

⚡ Over feeling that you were responsible. Somehow you are responsible for your father's death, even though you were hundreds of miles away at the time.

⚡ Over surviving when others did not. Your joy at surviving the boating accident conflicts with the fact that others did not survive.

Sadness

⚡ Over your painful loss. You are haunted with regrets over the loss of another person, a certain place, a part of yourself gone forever.

As we have seen, aftershock is a complicated phenomenon, one not easily defined or recognized. But it also has its positive effects; once you have suffered from a traumatic event, you begin to appreciate life and no longer put off your dreams. How many people decide to take that cruise after they have recovered from a heart attack? How many people found a better job and a better lifestyle after getting fired? How many people come through their crisis stronger and wiser and ready to take charge of their own lives?

The answer is quite a few. People *do* recover from aftershock— and find themselves happier and healthier than they ever were before. But before you can journey toward health, you need to discover the symptoms that have weighed you down. Only then can you get rid of your pain, once and for all. In the next chapter, I will be going over the various aftershock symptoms one by one.

AFTERSHOCK SYMPTOMS

One year after her minor car accident, June still can't get back in the car and drive to the market.

At last, at fifty-one, Sol finally scored his first hole in one. He was shaking hands with his caddy, grinning from ear to ear, when he collapsed and died from a sudden, acute heart attack. Three months later the caddy complains of severe chest pains, pains that according to his doctor have no physical basis.

Jeff lost Benny, his Irish Setter, six months ago. He still keeps Benny's leash on the door and his bowl of water filled. He claims he hears Benny barking just before he falls asleep.

Screaming, "No, not me too!" Amy woke up from intense nightmares four weeks after her boss was fired in a merger and she got his job.

After witnessing a holdup in a grocery store, Chris became numb and withdrawn. One day he stopped talking completely. He hasn't spoken in six months.

From anxiety to severe depression, from hallucinations to fatal heart attacks, the symptoms of aftershock can hurt. But there is a positive side.

QUAE NOCENT, DOCENT

"Those things that hurt, also teach." It's an ancient Roman proverb that is as true today as when it was first said in the forum. Your reactions to a crisis might be less severe than in these extreme examples, but even one sleepless night, one bout of anxiety, one day of depression is one moment more of pain you should not have to suffer. Your feelings, your physical health, and your body's chemistry all give clues to your well-being and peace of mind. Listen to your thoughts and your body. Before you can learn from your traumatic experiences you must recognize and interpret your symptoms. There is no better teacher than yourself.

ALL SYSTEMS GO

A woman who's cleaning her house night and day might be a fanatic about cleanliness, unless she had just lost her husband. A man who hasn't had a decent night's sleep in months might be suffering stress from working too hard, unless he has been laid off. A teenager who has stopped eating might be considered an anorexic, unless she has just had an unpleasant sexual experience. The symptoms of aftershock only *appear* to be signs of other disorders. What distinguishes aftershock symptoms from those of the others is the fact that they always begin *after* a traumatic event. Personal histories, neurotic impulses, stress and other variables might make you more susceptible to aftershock, but it's the trauma that makes its symptoms grow.

If you have recently had a traumatic experience, you might be experiencing some of the aftershock symptoms without realizing it. Before I go over each symptom in detail, take a moment to do this quiz. Based on checklists therapists use to diagnose their patients, it will help you identify and recognize aftershock in yourself and in those around you.

Think about your life before and after the crisis. Place a checkmark next to any statement that applied to you before the event. Then place an X next to any statement that applies to you now. This will help determine whether your symptoms are a sign of a different disorder or a result of the crisis—and an aftershock condition.

PSYCHOLOGICAL SHOCK

1. I'm afraid to leave the house.
2. I can't get into my car.
3. I have an anxiety attack before going to my office.
4. I don't want anyone to touch me.
5. I'm worried all the time.
6. I wake up depressed every morning.
7. I can't fall asleep.
8. I have terrifying nightmares almost every night.
9. I'm very restless.
10. I'll read something over and over again and still not understand it.
11. I can't remember simple things.
12. My performance at work is off.
13. No one understands me.
14. I feel insecure around my friends.
15. I've become very fatalistic—and I can't help but feel that nothing will ever work out right.
16. I've developed a phobia.
17. I'm so wired.
18. Loud noises really bother me.
19. I start crying at the drop of a hat.
20. I can't get out of bed.
21. I have no desire to go out and have a good time.
22. I'm scared of getting a physical examination.
23. All I want to do is sleep.
24. I've started yelling at everyone at work.
25. I'm uncomfortable in crowds.
26. I have trouble expressing my feelings.
27. I think a lot about death.
28. I'm scared I might commit suicide.
29. I feel like a different person.

PHYSICAL SHOCK

1	I feel weak all over.
2	I get cold sweats when I sleep.
3	I have frequent headaches.
4	My hands shake.
5	I've lost weight.
6	All I want to do is eat.
7	I have ringing in my ears.
8	I get acid indigestion often.
9	I have shortness of breath.
10	My head feels clogged.
11	I've been smoking more and more.
12	I drink alone—and too often.
13	I need a tranquilizer to calm my nerves.
14	My heart beats too fast.
15	I have lost my appetite.
16	I hear voices.
17	I see visions.
18	My skin feels prickly.
19	My eyesight is blurry.
20	My joints ache.
21	I get frequent sore throats.
22	I'm nauseated.
23	I need to go to the bathroom frequently.
24	There's a tightness in my chest.
25	I have no interest in sex.
26	I feel slow—in my thoughts, in my actions, in making decisions.

If you have put X's by many of these statements, you could be suffering from aftershock. Of course, a complete physical examination must be made to make sure that your symptoms are not related to an organic disorder. But if you have recently gotten a clean bill of health from your physician, you might need therapeutic treatment.

GROWING PAINS

As I mentioned earlier, it's normal to have emotional outbursts and a period of denial right after a trauma. In fact it's important that you go through a catharsis; your body and your mind need release. But stable individuals who have suffered through a stressful life event will soon after find relief. Once the shock has worn off, they will be pleased that they were saved. They might get the shakes; they might have restless nights. But eventually they will be thankful they have survived intact. The trauma will be put away and they will go on with their lives. There may be times when it is remembered—a bad night's sleep, a flash of memory—but it will not interfere with daily routines.

Take John Connally. At one time, he was one of the most powerful citizens in Texas—and in the White House. He was worth millions, but he lost it all. Yet he has appeared on *Sixty Minutes* in good humor, accepting his situation and in his seventies recognizing his mistakes and going forward.

Normal responses to a traumatic crisis wear off, usually in four to six weeks. The nightmares, the insomnia, and the anxiety disappear. It's the symptoms that crop up weeks, months or even years later that cause problems.

ACUTE DISTRESS

In people suffering from aftershock, relief never comes. Instead, its victims often begin obsessing about the traumatic event. A person who has survived a terrible car accident and now suffers from aftershock will concentrate on how he or she might have been killed, instead of the fact she's alive and well.

This works with positive stress too. The woman who received her boss's job when he got fired was afraid she would get fired too, instead of enjoying the promotion.

ONE KIND OF AFTERSHOCK

When symptoms crop up within six months of the trauma, I call it acute aftershock. Anxiety stays at a high level; there is no release. The trauma becomes the focal point of the victim's life.

Alicia had been married for fifteen years. She thought she had a terrific marriage; her friends envied her wedded bliss. "Oh," Alicia would tell them with a shrug and a smile, "I work at it." And she did, too. While Rob was in medical school, Alicia took a job in a local bank as a secretary. Her employer offered to pay her way through business school, but she declined. There wouldn't be time to be with Rob and take care of the grocery shopping, the dry cleaning, the cooking and the daily errands. Rob's career came first. There would be time later for Alicia.

But that time never came. Instead, Rob graduated from school and eventually established a flourishing practice. Alicia quit her job at the bank and became a full-time mother. Even then, at night, she would dream of going back to school. She was fully prepared to do so when the boys were old enough. Rob supported her; he told her he was proud of her. In fact, he suggested she start school whenever she chose. Alicia always said later, when the kids were older. Rob readily agreed.

Then one day, while Alicia was putting away some clothes in Rob's drawer, she noticed some credit card receipts from a trip to Paris, one she never took with Rob. When Alicia confronted him, Rob broke down. He told her that he had been having an affair with a nurse in the office. It had been going on for years and Rob loved the woman. Rob was glad it had come out. He wanted a divorce.

At first, Alicia tried to pretend all was well. She wanted an amicable divorce. She and Rob were adults; there were the children to consider. But when the divorce papers came through, she broke down and cried. The full impact of the last fifteen years hit her hard. Alicia was devastated. She started to grow angry; she fired the family friend representing her and hired a legal "Young Turk." She wanted retribution; she wanted payback.

Soon her life was nothing but divorce. That was all Alicia talked about with her friends, with her family, with her lawyer. She started to drink. Her hands shook. She stopped taking care of herself in the meticulous way she always had. She lost interest in her house, her sons, her life. Eventually, even her most sympathetic friends stopped calling.

The fact was that Alicia became too self-centered, too involved in herself and the divorce. Alicia suffered from acute aftershock.

Acute aftershock victims suffer from a snowballing effect. The more they think about the trauma, the more anxious they feel. The more anxious they feel, the more they think about the trauma.

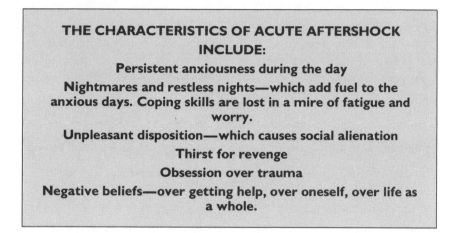

THE CHARACTERISTICS OF ACUTE AFTERSHOCK INCLUDE:

Persistent anxiousness during the day

Nightmares and restless nights—which add fuel to the anxious days. Coping skills are lost in a mire of fatigue and worry.

Unpleasant disposition—which causes social alienation

Thirst for revenge

Obsession over trauma

Negative beliefs—over getting help, over oneself, over life as a whole.

When symptoms persist for over six months, acute aftershock becomes chronic.

CHRONIC AFTERSHOCK

Remember Rosemarie and the dead cockroach? She is a prime example of a chronic aftershock victim. Her first response was normal, but it soon developed into an acute stage, complete with obsessions about cockroaches and food. The more Rosemarie worried, the more her anxiety stayed at a high level and the more her stress-related physical ailments continued. Soon she developed cold after cold, became convinced she had developed a disease from eating the tainted muffin, and even began to feel some distressing physical symptoms. Several months later, she had almost forgotten the initial trauma. It was buried under a mass of physical worries.

And that is the main characteristic of chronic aftershock. Attention switches to the body, especially when medical professionals give the victim a clean bill of health. Instead of believing the doctor, instead of seeking psychological help, chronic victims become convinced that people think they are going crazy. They get third, fourth, even fifth, opinions, hoping against hope they will feel the way they felt before the trauma. Victims may turn to alcohol and drugs during the acute stage to seek release, but when their condition turns chronic, substance abuse becomes a problem in and of itself. Depression settles in and suicide is uppermost in their minds.

Rather than being fixated on the crisis, a chronic aftershock victim is fixated on its consequences. And the more chronic a condition becomes, the less a victim is inclined to seek psychiatric help. Treatment is delayed, sometimes until it is too late.

HE WHO HESITATES IS LOST

The *DSM-III-R* classifies symptoms of PTSD that do not appear for six months or longer following trauma as delayed PTSD. Though useful to lawyers filing damage suits, delayed PTSD is shrouded in controversy.

The causes for delayed PTSD include extreme repression of the painful event, with defense mechanisms so efficient that they have helped put the trauma out of the victim's mind. But more times than not it is the treatment that has been delayed—not the response. In reality, a victim of delayed PTSD is a victim of chronic aftershock who has waited to seek help or who has been forced to wait to seek help.

A case in point is the Vietnam vet. The delayed reaction seemingly seen in so many returned soldiers was in actuality the delayed reaction of the government in setting up aid for PTSD sufferers. The Vietnam vets had had PTSD a long time before the government recognized it for what it was.

EARLY SIGNS

These are the symptoms of aftershock that appear first. They might be seen in relatively stable people within four to six weeks after a trauma —as in someone who experiences the death of a loved one, mourns, then gets on with life—or in victims of acute aftershock in its early stages.

1. Lack of sleep. You have just received a promotion and you are anxious. Every time you put your head on the pillow, you start thinking about the job: your strategies, your coworkers, your new manager. You are afraid they will "find you out" and fire you. This lack of sleep makes you more anxious during the day.

2. Jumpiness and increased irritability. If you are not getting a good night's sleep, you are just not going to cope as well during the day. When Janice became a new mother, she didn't glow, she glowered. She was so tired and apprehensive that she would do the wrong thing, she couldn't relax.

3. Nightmares. Freud once said that the repeating of a trauma, whether in dreams or in life, was a way of attempting to get it right, to regain mastery over a situation. Nightmares also keep the crisis very much alive.

4. Numbness. This is a way of denying the trauma, of desensitizing yourself to the crisis. In fact, victims of accidents who suffered amnesia—the ultimate numbness—actually had less aftershock symptoms than people who were in a waking state. They couldn't constantly replay the event in their minds.

5. Depression. In 1962, a study by David Mechanic of graduate students about to take their qualifying exams found that the students displayed varying symptoms of strain, from allergies to nausea, from hyperventilation to fatalism, as the day and hour of the exam drew near. One student complained: "Lately, I've been feeling real depressed. I don't feel that I know anything. I just feel so mentally defective, like what I have done goes into one ear and out the other. . . . I'm just sort of tired of the whole business. I'm tired of studying. I'm tired of school. I'm just tired . . ." As with these students, depression sets in because of that crucial element of trauma, lack of control. If one feels helpless, or in someone else's power, it's easy to feel down.

6. Impulsive, erratic behavior. A plane crash occurred down the block from Mrs. L's house. She heard the noises; she could see the burst of flames. She opened her screen door and peered outside. She then went into the bedroom, pulled off the sheets and proceeded to do a laundry.

When these symptoms persist, they become chronic. They also become more serious and more difficult to treat.

HEAVY METTLE

Think of approaching winter. You are wearing a light jacket; the air starts to chill. You pile on a sweater and you are still not warm. You try a few more sweaters, a heavy coat, a scarf, and hat. But the winds keep blowing; you can't get warm. And you are so encumbered by your layers of clothes that you can barely move. The extra weight is getting you down.

Aftershock is cumulative. The longer your acute symptoms persist, the more chronic—and serious—they become. Soon you are so entrenched in your "layers" of symptoms that the symptoms themselves become the problem, the initial activating trauma all but forgotten.

SEVERE DEPRESSION

Greg had gotten used to a good lifestyle. The golden boy in his investment house, he had displayed his business acumen in smart buying and selling. He didn't use insider tips, but he did keep his finger on the stock market pulse. Unfortunately for Greg, others in his company, including his best friend Peter, were not as ethical. The scandal so destroyed Peter that he committed suicide. Many other friends lost their jobs and their reputations. The firm was threatened with bankruptcy. Greg held on to his job but he had to take a tremendous cut in salary. That, coupled with his friend's disgrace and with his own losses in the market, made him face a difficult reality. Instead of the good life, he had to learn to tighten his belt. At first he maintained a stoic attitude. But as the weeks went by, it got harder and harder. The worst week was when he had to sell his apartment—at a loss. Things began to fall apart. Six weeks after the initial crisis, he became depressed. Now, six months later, his depression has gone from bad to worse. He hasn't looked for a job. He hasn't gone out with anyone. His initial depression has become an albatross, a disease unto itself. Without proper treatment, it will get worse.

PHOBIAS

Greg has developed a fear of money. He is terrified to let it go. He counts his change at night; once he went into a panic when he discovered that he had a Canadian penny. He barters at the cash register of his local grocery store. Another man, who had been involved in a car crash, begins to tremble if he has to get into a car. A woman who survived a flood gets cold sweats every time it starts to rain. And Rosemarie screams when she sees a bug. These individuals are all suffering from unreasonable fears or phobias, as a direct result of their aftershock.

PANIC ATTACKS

This particular Monday, Greg awakened around 6:30, the time he used to get up when he had had a job. He stretched, shaved, and showered just like the old days. He checked his closet and took out his cashmere suit. Greg was going on a job interview and he wanted to look sharp. He turned on the *Today* show while he poured some coffee. He was whistling. This was going to be it. The show switched to a commercial; a group of carefree, good-looking young adults were sharing a soda. Greg sipped his coffee; he was aimlessly watching the tube. Suddenly Greg started to cry. He wiped his nose on his good cashmere suit. His hands began to shake and he had to undo his tie. He couldn't breathe. He knew he was going to die.

Panic attacks become more severe the longer aftershock symptoms persist. As Greg can attest, the slightest stimulus from the environment can set an attack in motion. There is no thought between stimulus and response; the body responds automatically—the "fight or flight" phenomenon I talked about in Chapter Three.

Interestingly, community-wide disasters, such as a flood or a hurricane, result in more anxiety attacks than combat. A study of Mt. St. Helens disaster victims found at least 83 percent of them exhibiting apprehension, trouble concentrating, and hyperactivity—all signs of panic and anxiety. Only 63 percent of combat war veterans showed trouble concentrating. Only 50 percent were apprehensive. And only 38 percent of the combat war veterans displayed hyperactive symptoms.

SEXUAL DYSFUNCTION

The last thing now on Greg's mind was sex. He could barely get dressed in the morning, let alone perform. His girlfriend had been coming by every day after work, trying to get Greg to eat, to show some animation. Finally, she gave up. Puzzled, she told Greg he needed help, that she would be there if he needed her, but for now there was nothing else she could do. She too had needs. Greg just lay sprawled on his couch; he remained unresponsive. Like his depression, his sexual impotence had become a problem unto itself.

MORE AND MORE WITHDRAWAL FROM THE WORLD

A typical characteristic of chronic aftershock is avoidance—of family, of friends. A victim becomes unemotional and cold, cutting off all ties of support. And the more withdrawn he or she gets, the more people *want* to stay away—a double-edged sword of despair.

When Greg began to withdraw from his girlfriend, his family, and his friends, they tried to reason with him. But Greg would only sit there nodding his head, muttering "Leave me alone." They eventually did.

HALLUCINATIONS AND VIVID FLASHBACKS

Remember the network theory of PTSD I discussed in the previous chapter? The traumatic experience "etching" a passageway through the brain—and reactivating when triggered by an environmental stimulus? It's a very real, very immediate re-experiencing of the trauma.

Ask Greg. His trauma came back with the sights and sounds of the trading floor on the local news. It came back every time he looked at the spot where his sofa had been before he had sold it to pay the rent. It came back every day when the early morning light hit his bed, so strong, so sweet, he wanted to cry in pain.

One study that sought to elicit recollection from Vietnam combat veterans found there is a real reliving of the trauma in an aftershock victim's mind. Sixty-one percent of the subjects did more than recollect. In their minds they went back to the jungles of Southeast Asia. Skin conductance went up; heartbeat grew rapidly faster; flashbacks were extremely visual and dynamic. And another study, comparing eight Vietnam vets who suffered from PTSD with Vietnam vets who had no symptoms of PTSD, found that showing just fifteen minutes of the movie *Platoon* would evoke dramatic physiologic responses in the vets with PTSD—as if they were actually experiencing the war again— but not in those vets who did not have the condition.

DRUG ABUSE AND ALCOHOLISM

Greg was in such torment that he needed a release. He wasn't willing to go to a therapist; he was convinced his problems were physical. After all, how could his sleepless nights, his panic attacks, and his endless fatigue stem from a cut in pay? How could an event that not only happened six months ago, but that (if he said so himself) he had handled quite well, be the cause? A drink made him feel better. A Valium calmed his nerves. Another drink and another Valium were even better. They soothed his spirits, or so he thought.

In reality, drugs and alcohol cloud the issues. They cover up a problem instead of helping us overcome it, so the problem is never resolved or integrated into the person's mind. Suddenly Greg no longer had the problem of his aftershock. He had two more, alcohol and drug abuse.

ANTISOCIAL BEHAVIOR

It's a deadly cycle of self-destruction: The more you feel the world rejects you, the angrier you become. The angrier you become, the more you lash out. The more you lash out, the more you lose touch with reality. The more you lose touch with reality, the more you feel the world rejects you.

Take Greg. A few nights after a night of heavy drinking he took a cab to his girlfriend's apartment house and buzzed up. There was no answer. He buzzed again and continued to buzz. He started to yell, ran outside, grabbed a rock, and tried to break her window. He smashed a neighbor's first-floor apartment window instead.

Greg was angry and he lashed out at whoever was near. A Vietnam vet will take a fighting stance when he hears a loud noise. A violent-crime victim will open the door with a gun in his hand.

A way of acting out intense feelings, antisocial behavior is seen more in men than women. It may be more socially acceptable for women to become hysterical, or overanxious. Cultural conditioning dies hard. Even with as much progress as we have made in the past decades, men will still tend to react to trauma by aggressively lashing out at the outside world; women will react in a more internal fashion.

MENTAL BREAKDOWNS LEADING TO HOSPITALIZATION

Greg's outburst on the city streets ultimately became his salvation; he had been on a downward spiral with no end in sight. The police had picked him up and kept him overnight for disturbing the peace. When his parents bailed him out, they refused to hear his rationalizations. They brought him to a psychiatrist who, after exhaustive tests to determine Greg's disorder, admitted him to a hospital for treatment.

Greg had had a mental breakdown, but today he is on his way to complete recovery. He no longer drinks; he has moved to a smaller town with a better quality of life; he has started his own consulting firm and is about to marry the woman who sold him his new house. He is taking a course in art history at the local college, because, as he tells it, "Life is too short to wait to do the things I always wanted to do."

SUICIDE

Greg was lucky. Some people don't get help before it's too late. An esteemed colleague of mine, author and journalist Walter Reich, points out that the words "homicide," "suicide," and "decide" all end with *cide*, from the Latin word meaning to kill. In essence, "decide" means to kill off your options. But only one of the three words gives birth to hope. If you must choose from among the three, *decide* now to get help —before it is too late.

LET'S GET PHYSICAL

In addition to the psychological symptoms of aftershock, there are physical reactions as well, the biological and chemical reactions that go on in your body to create more stress, that provide the fuel for even more emotional distress.

Studies indicate that people's emotional states influence their sense of physical well-being. People in poor physical health

⚡ Are frequently depressed
⚡ Feel neglected

� Have low morale
✗ Feel alienated
✗ Are unsatisfied with life

Stress—and its resulting distress—are the keys to the amount of pain you feel. Pain is subjective. Just as the magnitude of a trauma has no bearing on the way you will react, the damage done your body in an accident has no relationship to the degree of discomfort you will feel. Both your reaction and your pain are directly related to the anxiety you have at the time of the traumatic event.

Greg's stress levels were high at the time of the stock market crash. They continued to escalate causing him a great deal of physical pain. He couldn't breathe. He was nauseated. When he kicked his sofa at one point in frustration, the jolt of pain he felt was excruciating. He had no tolerance for even the slightest tension headache.

Though our tolerance for pain is based on our anxiety, it is our backgrounds that motivate our ways of handling pain. A study conducted in 1952 of ethnic groups and pain discovered that Jews and Italians are much more emotional about their pain than white-Anglo-Saxon-Protestants. Jews are more concerned with the significance of their pain on their future, whereas Italians are interested in more immediate relief. WASPs try to be stoic and objective, and the Irish have been brought up to deny their pain exists.

Popular psychologists tell their patients to feel the pain. I take that one step further. Feel the pain—and understand it. Understand why you are feeling pain, and perhaps most important, understand that this pain is not permanent; it can and will go away with treatment. Recognizing the physical effects of aftershock will not only help reduce the anxiety you are experiencing but can also save your life.

I. BRAIN DYSFUNCTION

Anxiety is all in your head—literally. The chemicals that surge through your brain's passageways constrict and open blood vessels; they stimulate motor controls and heartbeat; they dictate your emotions by unleashing mood-altering hormones into your system; they activate the "running tapes" of memory stored in different parts of your brain.

To be specific:

⟋ Massive noradrenergic (hormonal) stimulation of the part of the brain called the locus ceruleus and the hippocampus keeps those vivid flashbacks and fragments alive.

⟋ The depletion of the neurochemicals norepinephrene (NE) and dopamine, synthesized by the brain in times of unavoidable shock, causes diminished motivation, numbness, fatigue, inability to work, and alienation from others. NE's synthesis is "etched" on the brain, triggering the same debilitating reactions in subsequent minor and avoidable shocks.

⟋ The unleashed adrenaline surge found in the constant "fight or flight" effect of aftershock acts as an engine in the brain to keep you traumatized.

2. IRREGULAR HEARTBEATS

Studies show that war veterans having experienced a traumatic event show an erratic heartbeat with no apparent physical cause. This irregular rhythm throws off breathing, causes hyperventilation, creates the feeling of having a heart attack, and triggers those ubiquitous panic attacks.

3. INCREASED RATE IN BLOOD PRESSURE AND HEART RATE

Ten days after President Kennedy's assassination, the twenty-seven-year-old army captain in charge of his ceremonial funeral procession died of cardiac irregularity and acute congestion, positive proof that the physical symptoms of aftershock must be watched and checked. More proof: A study done by Dr. C. M. Parkes and colleagues found a higher rate of heart attack death in grieving spouses during the six months after they suffered their loss.

4. CLAMMY SKIN

The expression "It made my skin crawl" is more fact than fancy. In a branch of medicine called psychophysiology they actually determine heart rate and skin conductance. During a trauma, blood rushes through your system; adrenaline surges through your body. You feel sweaty, cold, and clammy, all at the same time. War veterans, reliving the trauma of combat when combat scripts were read to them, experienced rapid heartbeat and clammy skin.

5. NUMB FEELING

That tingling feeling in your fingers and toes, the sensation of sleep-walking, that all-encompassing numb feeling, all have a physical cause that has nothing to do with grade-B zombie movies. When you experience a shock, the adrenal glands' cortex slackens its activity, which makes you feel numb.

In fact, the out-of-body experiences described by people after a traumatic event are really a product of this low cortical activity, with its characteristic numbness and disassociation. A tragic example comes from women who have been raped. Many report a profound disassociation during the crime, as if they are floating above their own bodies detached from their attacker.

Numb feelings also come from extreme denial, when the denial and intrusive stages of aftershock (which I discussed in Chapter Three) take on problematic proportions. Numbness is an unnatural overcontrol, just as the repetitions of the stressful event in the form of nightmares, intrusive thoughts, and flashbacks are seen as defensive *under*control—or failure. Both might be present. A woman being raped might deny the act itself, but she will replay the moment the attacker crept into her bedroom window.

6. IMMUNE SYSTEM EFFECTS

It's a proven fact: stress reduces our resistance. Combat soldiers catch colds. Many doctors now believe that stress may play an important role in weakening our immune system and making it vulnerable to diseases such as cancer and Epstein-Barr virus (sometimes called chronic mononucleosis) that attack the immune system.

A case in point is a study done by Dr. Janice K. Kiecolt-Glaser and Dr. Ronald Glaser. They observed seventy-five first-year medical students and found a significant drop in their bodies' natural killer-cell activity levels during finals. Similarly, Dr. Steven J. Schleifer examined fifteen husbands whose wives died from breast cancer and found immune system chemicals significantly lowered in all of them for two months following the deaths. Two years later, after time had done its healing, the men's levels were back to normal.

Whether physical or psychological, it's crucial to diagnose aftershock correctly and to make certain its symptoms are not indicative of other diseases. It can make all the difference between treatment that is ineffectual and treatment that brings good health.

DIFFERENT STROKES

Because I am a specialist in emergency psychiatry, the first time I meet a new patient, he or she is usually in a crisis state. Time is of the essence to reduce any life-threatening symptoms. I have seen suicidal teenagers rushed in on gurneys, hysterical men and women in highly agitated states, victims of heart attacks, unconscious drug abusers, people in the throes of such profound depression that they are catatonic, and more. Once I have administered life-saving procedures, I focus on diagnosing their problem and on conducting the proper tests that will help me discover the illness inside and determine the best methods of therapy—both pharmaceutical and psychological. These tests include blood tests and psychological tests, EEGs and CAT scans, complete physicals and stress evaluations.

The *one* element that separates my aftershock patients from others is the trauma. Period. If they display its symptoms without having had a traumatic event, I look elsewhere, from general anxiety to brain tumors. If their symptoms have been diagnosed since childhood, I must determine if they were intensified by the traumatic event or an omnipresent on-going condition. If they have been a part of a patient's "standard operating procedure," I can rule out aftershock.

Further, I must determine if their crisis situation is stable, if they are going through the normal stages of emotions anyone would experi-

---

AFTERSHOCK CAN LOOK LIKE:
Normal guilt and sadness resulting from a loss
Manic-depression
Schizophrenia
Compulsive-obsessive disorders
Physical illness
General anxiety and depression

ence after a trauma, and if their coping skills are intact. If so, time can heal most of their wounds and intensive therapy is not needed.

A wide range of psychiatric conditions, from manic-depression to schizophrenia, from obsessive-compulsive disorders to normal guilt—any one of these illnesses can cause patients to have hallucinations, to be depressed and out of sorts, to alienate themselves from the world. But always, with aftershock, there is the trauma: the battery, the starter, and the fertilizer.

The treatment for aftershock varies from individual to individual. In Part III, I will go over the entire therapy process from beginning to the healthful and hopeful end.

Why is it that some people develop aftershock and others don't? Who is at risk? Before we go on to treatment, let's see who aftershock strikes—and why.

WHO IS AT RISK?

L ISTEN TO THIS PATIENT TALKING DURING AN ACTUAL session with
myself and my colleague Dr. Glicksman:

> QUESTION: If you were . . . talking to someone like ourselves,
> someone who does crisis intervention, what advice would you
> give? . . . Have you learned anything through your [traumatic]
> experience?
> PATIENT: I really believe it's a matter of whether you are built
> fearless or you are built fearful mentally. You know the guys who
> go in and charge during the war and risk their lives without
> thinking, even if they have not been taking any bromide or any
> alcohol and some others will just tremble because it's just a mat-
> ter of mental buildup and there is no courage. Some people are
> courageous and some are not that courageous.

This man, a victim of an elevator crash, was speaking from the
depths of experience, from a firsthand view of the fine line between life

and death. As he plunged into the darkness of the elevator shaft, his thoughts were on survival, not on acts of courage or fearlessness. He was operating on a primal level, just as we all do when faced with a sudden traumatic event.

But as he slowly regained consciousness in his hospital bed, as the full impact of the accident hit him, this man continued to act with strength. Why? Why did he turn out healthy—and wiser—while others with similar experiences find themselves in the torturous throes of aftershock? Some of the answer lies in the victim's emotional state at the time of the trauma. As we discovered in Chapter Three, the more anxiety and stress you are feeling at that time, the better your chances of getting aftershock. The rest of the equation, as the wizard told Dorothy, lies within your own backyard.

BLOOD IS THICKER THAN WATER

Some of us are born with an innate strength. Others learn courage and the value of support. Still others are brought up scared, with fears that never go away.

Environment and heredity: Our family tree dictates our height, intelligence, and eye color; its locale affects our personality and value system. Even as we focus on our present and make far-reaching plans, our backgrounds continue to operate behind the scenes, consciously or unconsciously influencing our lives. Our backgrounds provide the ingredients for predictability, guiding us in whom we marry, where we live, how we think—and whether or not we might get aftershock.

Though it's a proven fact that anyone will succumb to aftershock if a life event is traumatic enough, there are certain conditions, values, and beliefs that will either help us pass through a crisis unscathed and resilient or make aftershock a reality.

FAMILY TIES

Anxiety runs in families and so does susceptibility to aftershock. A study done by Dr. R. G. McInnes as far back as 1937 concluded that only 8.3 percent of the siblings of nonanxious parents developed anxiety disorders themselves. But when only one parent had a history of anxiety, the figure rose to 26.5 percent. Another study in 1980, found that 41 percent of the relatives in anxious families had a predilection for anxiety—as opposed to only 8 percent of the relatives from nonanxious families.

When Dr. C. B. Scrignar studied ten victims of a minor gas leak accident in a factory, he discovered that six workers regained their health after a few weeks. The other four, though they too received a clean bill of health, developed symptoms of aftershock, ranging from insomnia and anxiety to nightmares and respiratory ailments. In subsequent interviews with the victims, Dr. Scrignar learned that the six completely recovered workers grew up in stable families while the "aftershock four" grew up in families fraught with worry or in broken homes. They had also suffered, as children and young adults, more colds, stomach ailments, and other illnesses that can be caused or aggravated by anxiety, than the recovered workers.

If you come from a troubled family or have a history of panic attacks either in your adolescence or young adulthood, your anxiety could already be operating at a high level, increasing the possibility of aftershock following a traumatic event.

LEAVING THE NEST

June's parents had always wanted to send her to summer camp to enjoy the great outdoors as they had at her age. Throughout the fall and winter they told her all about the group activities and sports she would enjoy, the friends she would meet, and the memories she would treasure. But June didn't share their enthusiasm. All she wanted was to stay home and play with her friends in the neighborhood. Her parents chalked up her hesitation to first-time jitters. After all, any twelve-year-old girl should jump at the chance to go to sleepaway camp.

When June said good-bye to her parents at the bus, she was crying and sniffling. Unfortunately she didn't stop. For two weeks she stayed in her bunk; she refused to play with the other children, and she cried herself to sleep every night. Finally the camp director called her parents. They tried to reason with her on the phone, urging her to give camp a chance. A week later June went home.

What might have been a minor trauma to someone else was a major event in June's life. That first separation anxiety followed her through her adult years, preventing her from going to an out-of-state college and marrying a man that she loved.

More serious separation anxiety may occur in children from divorced homes and in alcoholic families. A test done on children of alcoholics by Professor Carlene Riccelli at the University of Massachusetts showed that adult children of alcoholics have problems with intimate relationships; they often lack the capacity for carefree fun and a high proportion of them tend to take themselves too seriously.

A history of separation anxiety almost guarantees an aftershock reaction to trauma.

THE PRODIGAL SON

Truancy, stealing, lying, running away, fighting, sexual promiscuity, drug abuse, bad grades—these behavioral problems read like a parent's worst nightmare come true. In a study done of PTSD in the general population, it was discovered that 29 percent of the people who suffered from aftershock had had more than four of these problems as a child. Maladjusted children who do not work through their problems later on in therapy almost always react to trauma with aftershock symptoms.

AN UNWELCOME GUEST

We all have ingrained beliefs, some of them more irrational than others. But steadfast beliefs like these: "Wishing makes it so," "My bad thoughts can hurt others," "I need to be loved beyond all else," and "I need love to survive" open the door to aftershock and invite it in to stay. These thoughts indicate not only an inflated view of one's power but also a belief that one's self-esteem must be bestowed on one by another's love.

If you share these beliefs, they will not only reinforce the guilt you feel after a trauma but will also make you feel: (1) a lack of control, (2) depressed and fearful, and (3) irrationally responsible for a stressful event. Remember those five PTSD emotions I wrote about in Chapter Three, those strong feelings of rage, worry, guilt, fear, and sadness that form a part and parcel of a shock's aftermath? These beliefs keep them fresh and strong.

And if you pair these ingrained beliefs with equally strong but contradictory values, your susceptibility to aftershock increases dramatically. A man who steadfastly believes in his marriage, but also dreams of having an affair, will be filled with anxiety and stress; he is an aftershock victim waiting for an event to happen.

THE "FELIX UNGER" SYNDROME

Every one knows at least one. Perhaps one is a member of your family or a friend or colleague at work. Maybe it's you. The perfectionist. The person who constantly tries to do the right thing no matter what, who feels he or she has failed if it rains on their parade, who can't take a compliment with a simple thank you, who never seems to slow down. Perfectionists leave themselves no room for failure, but since perfection is an impossible goal, they always find themselves falling short, and a cycle of perceived failure and poor self-image results. After a supposed failure, instead of setting more realistic goals and giving themselves credit for what they did accomplish, perfectionists browbeat themselves with reproaches like: "Next time I won't let that happen. . . . I can't believe I made that mistake! . . . How stupid of me! . . ." The result?: a bad self-image and a pervasive lack of confidence. And with these attitudes perfection becomes more unattainable still.

Always wanting to do the right thing is as harmful as the need to have everyone love you. Ingrained perfectionist attitudes and impossible goals create anxiety and traumatic aftershock.

THE DOOR IS ALWAYS LOCKED

John was meticulous. He religiously wrote his plans out every day in his Filofax planner, from waking up and showering to his twenty minutes of Johnny Carson before dozing off. He was a super financial analyst at a Fortune 500 company, respected by his peers and admired by his family. Seemingly perfect, John always kept his feelings locked up, never wanting to be a burden to anyone.

But when he fell in love with Allison, his whole world changed. Instead of numbers he pictured her. Instead of planning futures he planned his wedding day. Unfortunately, Allison did not reciprocate his affections. She went out with him for a few months, but despite his strong feelings for her he could not be spontaneous, he refused to open up. She broke off their relationship, and John went into a tailspin. He began to exhibit all the signs of aftershock, from depression to obsession-filled fantasies, from numbness to ambivalent aches and pains.

John's repressed feelings made him vulnerable to aftershock.

THE HEAD OF THE HOUSEHOLD

Control is a big issue in the 1980s. We try to control our working lives, our daily routines, our inner selves, our homes and our health. But some things we cannot control, especially a sudden, unexpected traumatic event. Studies indicate that the more control a person feels during a crisis, the less the negative impact of stress. Studies have also shown that people who feel they have at least some control over their environment are better able to adjust to stressful crises, perhaps by trying to find a way to repair the damage or to figure a way out of their situation.

But individuals who lack a sense of control develop what is called learned helplessness. These individuals, perceiving themselves as powerless and completely dependent on other forces for their survival, experience the full force of the stressful crisis. Unfortunately many aftershock situations exacerbate the feelings of powerlessness. Imagine being a passenger on a hijacked plane with a bomb-carrying terrorist on board, and you can see why this crisis is a likely precursor to aftershock.

A HOUSE UNITED

People need people. It's trite but true. Whether your social mix is found among family members or within a close circle of friends, the support, the kindness, and the understanding you receive—or don't receive—from them can make all the difference in whether or not you get aftershock after a traumatic event. The value of social support cannot be underestimated. It's an essential tool of both aftershock therapy and aftershock prevention.

THE FAMILY CIRCLE

The predilections I have outlined here can become a destructive self-prophecy: the more vulnerable you are to experiencing a traumatic crisis, the more vulnerable you will be to aftershock. If you are constantly worried about your marriage breaking up, your negativism can provide the wedge. If you constantly blame others at work for your own mistakes, you can lose your job. If you are in a dreamlike state, you could lose control of your car.

Remember Jim Ryun, the track star of the 1960s who would set world records in the mile but who never seemed to win a big race? Time and time again he would work himself up into such a nervous state that failure was almost automatic. During the 1968 Olympics, with the whole world watching, Ryun actually tripped during the race, finishing in a dismal time. It took years for him to recover from that letdown. He made a life-changing event even more traumatic.

In a similar vein is the story of a woman who had just lost her husband. She was so grief-stricken that a few months later, failing to pay attention while driving, she drove her car off the road and almost died in a near-fatal crash.

These are not examples of omens and witchcraft. Believe it or not, our negative thoughts can actually become so strong and so prevalent that we actually will traumatic events our way. We can allow them to happen.

But there is good news. We are not doomed to a lifetime of failure caused by our negative thoughts. With effort and patience, and with therapy if necessary, we can overcome our negativity. This means, not that we will never fail again, but rather that this time we will be able to learn from our failures and go on to greater successes. As Nietzche wrote: "What does not break makes one strong."

THE WELCOME MAT

Shortcomings can become strengths. Flaws can turn into assets. What you are today can bring you success in the future. Your individuality and your uniqueness have much to offer the world. The painter Edvard Munch said this forcefully in a letter he wrote to colleague K. E. Schreiner. Listen:

My art had its roots in my search for an explanation of life's inconsistencies. Why was I not like other people? Why was I born when I never asked to be? It was my rage at this injustice and my continual thinking about it that influenced all my art; these thoughts lay behind all my work and without them my art would have been completely different.

It was this difference that made him the great artist that he was, applauded and celebrated through the years. You too can make your differences work for you—and flourish.

All is not bleak. All that looks like potential causes for aftershock can be overcome. But before you can seek help and change your ways, you must first find knowledge—and understanding.

We have now learned exactly what aftershock is, and who is susceptible to its snare. In the next section, I will be going over specific traumas of the eighties to help you identify your personal pressure points. Only then can you learn to avoid the aftershock trap. Only then can you find hope and peace. Only then can you go on to therapy and prevention and the road to a better world for yourself and for those you love. Let's begin.

PART TWO:

THE
SHOCKING
EVENT

EVENTS THAT CAN SHAKE YOUR WORLD

6

IT IS THE ULTIMATE NIGHTMARE, A ROOM THAT holds your greatest fear and unleashes it to break you. For the characters in George Orwell's *1984*, it is the quintessential police-state device, a place that knows their innermost dread and waits, filled—sometimes with rats, sometimes merely with complete and total darkness—for them to enter.

Happily, our own 1984 has come and gone without Orwell's dark vision of the future. That fearful room is the stuff of science fiction after all. But everyone, even the calmest, most levelheaded person, has a breaking point that a trauma, or a series of traumas, can set off and bring on aftershock.

In the 1980s there are many such traumatic breaking points—some that change life for the better, some that make things worse—but all of them potential aftershock pitfalls.

A ROOM WITHOUT WALLS

The rules are different today. Japan is realizing the economic goals it had as an imperialistic enemy of the United States just forty years ago. Hitler's resort in the Bavarian alps has become a popular tourist spot. Foreign cars are being manufactured in America, then sold and touted as made in the USA. The British corporate giant, Saatchi & Saatchi, has taken over America's advertising world, buying out agency after agency along Madison Avenue. And the list goes on.

Fears and fraught with ambiguity. There are no perfect heroes, and evil is not confined to Orwell's dark room. The comfort of intimacy is threatened by AIDS. The reality of terrorism is in danger of coming closer to home. People are being more careful in their careers, in romance, in financial planning, and in every other aspect of life.

The world today is a complicated place, as we have seen here and in earlier chapters. But there is good news. Divorce rates might be up, but more and more people are getting married. Death might be more sudden and commonplace, but more and more people are having babies. The homeless are among us in larger and larger numbers, but so are the more affluent. Life in the eighties is more stressful, but we have more choices than we have ever had before.

Look around you and listen. The concepts of society are changing. National boundaries are slowly eroding, and with them prejudice and narrow thinking. There is more openness among nations, a global understanding that is eroding the desire for war and enlarging ever so slightly the possibilities of peace. Personally, professionally, and communally—the eighties bring both fearsome tidings and unlimited hope.

THE EIGHTIES SHAKEDOWN

Today's stressful, life-changing events can be divided into three groups:

✓ World and current events. These are the events that have a global impact and affect you in their wake. They include the unique trends in today's world—from war and epidemics to what the *DSM-III-R*, in its strict trauma definition, characterizes as "crimes outside the ordinary realm of experience."

✗ Personal events. Here are the stressful life events that can shake up your world, from the death of a loved one to the birth of your baby, from divorce to relocating to a new city, from marriage to getting everything you want—and still feeling empty.

✗ Fast-track stress. This category includes the events of corporate life: the promotions and the firings, the mergers and the retirements, the unsympathetic bosses, and the office politics.

The next three chapters will present the more common stressors in each of these worlds, the "pressure points" that can build up and affect you and the people around you. Based on newspaper headlines, mental-health professional checklists, trade journals, medical and scientific studies, and marketing trends, each trauma is pinpointed, good and bad, all-encompassing and relatively minor.

Each pressure point fits the definition of trauma discussed in Chapter Two. Some can happen suddenly and unexpectedly. Others may make you feel out-of-control. Still others are totally unfair, and leave you feeling powerless and angry. Each trauma, or pressure point, is divided by category. Running heads on each page provide easy access. A reader's encyclopedia, these entries are designed to be read and reread, simply glanced over, or explored with complete concentration. Lists, anecdotes, and self-help hints will help you pinpoint your personal pressure points. For each entry, you will find:

✗ A brief history
✗ Cited studies that signal it for aftershock
✗ Case histories of people who have suffered from this trauma

Browse through these traumatic pressure points. Think about them and see how many pertain to your world, keeping in mind these four ways a trauma can hurt:

✗ If the event happened to you personally
✗ If you only witnessed the event and you had nothing to do with it
✗ If the event happened to someone you love or someone you merely know

⚡ If you helped someone through the trauma as part of your job

Together we can learn from today, from the crises that are as much a part of life as the changing seasons, as sundown and sunup, as growing older and wiser. Together we can understand the life and times of the disease of the 1980s called aftershock. And together, armed with that understanding, we can turn hope—for today and for tomorrow—into reality.

CRIMES AGAINST NATURE:

W A R A N D V I O L E N C E

7

Homo sum; humani nil a me alienum puto. (I am human, I hold nothing human alien to me.)
—TERENCE

I will never be sure of anything again.
—SECOND OFFICER, R.M.S. TITANIC

AFTERSHOCK HAS BECOME BIG NEWS, A CONDITION compensable by law, an insanity defense in a world gone mad. A Vietnam vet who killed a man is acquitted. A man who lost his legs in a train accident is being sued by the three members of the train's crew for "intentional neglect and infliction of emotional distress." From hospitals to power plants, corporations and governmental agencies, all are feeling the whiplash of the eighties, the phenomenon that is a direct result of our violent times.

It is proof positive that global events have a direct impact on our lives. There is no way of turning our heads. The events explode onto our TV screens, shout from our newspaper columns, and find their way into the house next door, bringing us a message of violence, fear, and fast-moving change.

In her novel *The Accidental Tourist*, Ann Tyler writes about a man who makes his living by reducing the shock of travel for Americans who have to, rather than wish to, travel around the world. He happily writes guidebooks to where real milk can be found in England, where white bread can be purchased in Italy, where American-style motels can be found in France, making the world a more manageable, safer, and more controllable place for his readers.

But it is all illusion. The world is out of control, changing even as I write these words. And the only way we can stop this constant change from hurtling aftershock in our direction is to make choices that are right for us. Examining today's global traumas will help us make good decisions, for ourselves and for generations to come. Read on.

WAR

A mathematician once calculated that there has been the equivalent of only one full day of peace since life began. Motivated by man, executed by man, and won and lost by man, war is as much an institution as our postal service and our neighborhood schools; it is an integral part of our heritage and our legacy worldwide.

When World War I broke out in Europe, Freud was still a believer in man's sexual and life-affirming forces. By the eve of World War II he had modified his stance, having decided that man was driven by self-destructive urges.

War is by definition a "crime outside the ordinary realm of experience," a crisis that more times than not results in aftershock. In our century, we have seen not one but two world wars, one fast on the heels of the other. Prior to the first World War, people lived in comparative innocence; it was an age of possibilities, of frivolity and earnest hope. World War I sobered humankind, but World War II was even worse. Gone was the optimism; innocence was irrevocably destroyed. Movies like *The Best Years of Our Lives* brought home the realities of war-weary men and their adjustment to civilian life. Amidst the joy of winning, there were the clouding facts that American ex-POWs were dying at a faster rate than their fellow vets, that many war wives became widows, that many of the surviving vets suffered from shell shock, and that things would never be the same again.

> Renowned author James Clavell spent four years in a Japanese prison camp where fourteen out of every fifteen fellow inmates died. He was one of the lucky ones. He almost starved to death but he survived. Yet fifteen years later, he was still fighting the impulse to forage through garbage cans for food. Fifteen years later, he still kept a solitary can of sardines in his kitchen—just in case. It was a secret he never shared with anyone.

War stands alone as a stressful life-changing event. It is entirely man-made, but it is also anonymous. Therefore, there is no one person to blame for the changes at home or for the death and destruction. To single out anyone would be considered unpatriotic.

But as cruel as our century's wars were, they form a common bond, a community of players who had shared in what they believed to be a just cause. The Vietnam War was different. Since it is this war that has recently brought aftershock to our attention, it is fitting to begin this section with a focus on this conflict.

PRESSURE POINT ONE: VIETNAM VETS TEN YEARS LATER

"How many walking time bombs like me are walking around and so damn lost? They do not know if they are coming or going. . . . When I die, Vietnam will have a lot to do with it" (from Dr. C. B. Scrignar's book *Posttraumatic Stress Disorder: Diagnosis, Treatment, and Legal Issues*, Praeger, 1984).That is a Vietnam vet talking, an ex-Marine who has suffered the pain of aftershock with no release. In and out of Veterans Administration hospitals, suffering from alcoholism and drug abuse, his aftershock culminated in a crime. He took a hospital worker hostage at gunpoint for several hours.

This vet is not alone. Twenty-five percent of those who saw heavy combat have been involved in a criminal offense since their homecoming, and only 4 percent of those offenders had prior psychological problems. The rest of the vets' criminal activity was a direct result of after-shock.

The Vietnam experience was unique. It is only now, after the fact, that we can see the aftershock in its survivors. In *Military Medicine*, Richard D. Marciniak recounts the work of J. P. Wilson and G. E. Krauss, two doctors who found that 75 percent of the Vietnam vets who suffered from PTSD had more severe cases if:

⟋ They had a very intense combat experience—in terms of the amount of time they were exposed to danger and the sense of helplessness they felt;

⟋ They had highly stressful combat duties—including long-range reconnaissance, exploration of enemy tunnels, POW incarceration, and grave registration detail; or

⟋ They felt a great deal of psychological isolation during the first six months after coming home, with lack of support, discrimination, and an inability to resume their previous occupational, educational, or social activities.

The reality is exposed by Kim Heron in an article published in *The New York Times Magazine:* out of the 500,000 aftershock-afflicted Vets, 150,000 are so severely afflicted that without therapy or medication, they will never lead a normal life.

The Vietnam experience was even more intense for black Americans. Studies show that blacks had more aftershock symptoms than their white counterparts: Forty percent of all black Vietnam vets succumbed to PTSD as opposed to only 20 percent for whites, and 70 percent of the black vets who saw heavy combat developed aftershock.

The realities of war hit black soldiers especially hard. The percentage of blacks who enlisted equaled the percentage of blacks in the general population, and almost all of those enlisted men tended to view the military in a favorable way. In their eyes, the military offered career and financial opportunities they might never have otherwise received. The black vets were also better educated than their civilian counterparts, the direct opposite of the situation among whites. These intelligent, hopeful men came to Vietnam with enthusiasm and found themselves in a moral and ethical crisis. Instead of heading into battle against a powerful Communist foe, they were waging a war against an

"One two three four, what are we fighting for?" This was the question protestors shouted while their fellow Americans were battling for their lives in Southeast Asia. This ambivalence was just one of the reasons why the Vietnam War was so different. Here are more:

Recruits were younger and therefore less knowledgeable about life and more vulnerable to its shocks. The average soldier in Vietnam was nineteen, as opposed to twenty three in World War II and twenty-four in Korea.

There was no consistency. Every year was different in terms of the intensity of combat, the attitude of the troops, and the political atmosphere back in the States.

The government introduced the DERO—for date of expected return from overseas—for the first time. Designed to reduce psychological and emotional damage by reducing the time of combat duty, DEROs prescribed a twelve-month tour of duty schedule for each soldier. (Marines had a thirteen-month schedule.) Consequently, there was a continuous coming and going within battalions. Friendships were broken before they began. Buddies were constantly saying good-bye. Group support was almost nil.

Friendships were not kept up back home. Unlike the American Legion and the clubs and fraternities for veterans of previous wars, the Vietnam veterans had no social postwar sphere. The DEROs that kept friendship to a minimum during the war kept friendships from continuing at home, increasing the isolation and likelihood of getting aftershock.

The Vietnam War was a guerrilla war that Americans fought in an unfamiliar territory with an alien landscape—a war in which confusion and extreme conditions were inherent. There was no way to prepare for the shock of encounter with swamplands and jungles, and the resulting hardships.

impoverished nonwhite country. In many cases they found themselves identifying with the enemy they were sent to destroy.

Meanwhile, back in the States Martin Luther King was assassinated and black militancy was on the rise. The black vets were ostracized by other blacks, condemned for fighting in a "white man's imperialistic war." Add to this the ambivalent climate all the returning vets faced, and you have a perfect environment for aftershock to develop.

The families of Vietnam vets also had their brand of aftershock, and some are still living through their trauma. An estimated 2541 vets are still listed as missing in action. They might be dead, they might be suffering from amnesia, they might be languishing in a Vietnamese prison. For these families, every day brings a little hope and much despair. They cannot go through the natural grieving process nor can they definitely declare their sons and fathers dead.

And what of the families that were fortunate enough to have a homecoming? Think of the expectations, the long year of waiting, the open arms—and then the son, father, or brother turning out to be a stranger, emotionally depleted and confused. The result? Just when the veteran needs his family most—and they need him—none of them find satisfaction.

The sobering fact of this pressure point is that in spite of all the evidence, in spite of the varied problems, in spite of the government's responsibility to these vets, only sixteen VA hospitals across the country have PTSD facilities.

PRESSURE POINT TWO: OTHER SOLDIERS, OTHER LIVES

Aftershock is not exclusively an American war disease. Soldiers in other countries have also experienced PTSD—though not as severely as our own Vietnam vets. In general, other soldiers have less alienation and anger and less antisocial behavior and adjustment problems, because war, unfortunately, has historically been a greater part of their lives. In a study done at the Israeli army's Central Mental Health Clinic, Dr. Bernard Lerer and colleagues found that Israeli soldiers had a lower incidence of alcohol and drug misuse and rebounded from war faster than their American counterparts.

It makes sense. There is a limited term of duty in Israel, one month a year. Soldiers are more confident; they are more likely to believe in what they are fighting for, more likely to trust their commanders and their comrades. Public attitudes too are more supportive. Everyone, including women and children, feels a part of a common cause.

This was not always the case. During the 1973 Arab-Israeli War, there were a great many psychiatric casualties within hours of the first shots. This so disturbed the Israeli government that it adopted the American method of frontline treatment, a combination of sleep, food and water, and a chance for the soldier to recount his or her traumatic experiences. This treatment proved successful; the Israel Defense Force was able to send 60 percent of its soldiers back to combat within seventy-two hours.

PRESSURE POINT THREE: CHILDREN OF THE HOLOCAUST

Some traumas are so extreme that to put them into words is to minimize them, to exploit them, and to do a disservice to those who have been affected. Such is the Holocaust. It must always be remembered so it will not happen again.

But in today's Austria and Germany, young people want to put the tragedy behind them. They are resisting feeling guilt for something they personally did not do. Austria and its controversial president want to forget the past.

But how can you tell a camp survivor to forget? Like the defeated character Rod Steiger played in the film *The Pawnbroker*, it's almost impossible for many survivors to enjoy life or trust others. Their painful memories and survivor guilt combine to create a chronic hopelessness and anxiety, which they unintentionally pass on to their children.

The Holocaust has become a family problem. Take the example of Nina, the thirty-year-old daughter of parents who met in a concentration camp and married when the war was over. Nina has had difficulty in her adult life. She has never made many friends; she is shy and withdrawn. She was a "model" teenager and she still complies with her parents' wishes. When a man she had been seeing asked her to marry him, Nina said no. She couldn't bear to leave her parents. She was passed over for a promotion at work, because her employer felt she wouldn't do well with client contact. Nina wasn't living; she was consumed with guilt.

Nina's situation is not uncommon among children of Holocaust survivors. A study of thirty-six survivor families found that the children expressed the pain the parents have denied—with bad grades, identity and sexual problems, hypochrondria, and depression. Rather than adding to their parents' pain with even the mildest rebellion, they kept their feelings and emotions under wraps.

Children of Holocaust survivors are also understandably overprotected. But this smothering mantle adds to the subconscious pressure on the children to provide their parents with a release from pain, a reason for happiness, a meaning for lives that had been terribly traumatized. Further, many survivors' children come to symbolize the relatives who were destroyed by the Holocaust, and they live with the apprehension that their slightest action will reawaken the painful memories of those lost loved ones.

Unfortunately, the burdens these children feel are often made even heavier by the tension-filled atmosphere of their parents' bad marriage. In order to stop the grief and the anxiety they experienced in the camps, many of the survivors married too quickly, with little in common besides a shared history of death and destruction.

For children of the Holocaust, the traumas of their parents live on in inherited aftershock.

VIOLENT CRIMES

Besides war, there are other crimes that go beyond our human endurance. These are the private violations, the traumas that are sudden, unfair, and threatening. These are the traumas of violence directed at the individual.

PRESSURE POINT FOUR: CRY RAPE!

A supreme violation, the trauma of rape unleashes waves of aftershock behavior. Think about it: Rape turns an act of intimacy and love into a terrifying defilement. Coupled with its inherent traumatizing fear of death is guilt—that subtle, insidious suspicion that somehow the victim let it happen. This has been compounded in the past by our judicial system, with judges erroneously believing that the victim invited the attack. A case in point involved a woman who had been raped by four men in a pool hall. As she sat in court one of the men's attorneys shifted the blame to her, claiming "she asked for it" by dressing provocatively.

But we have come a long way. In the *State of Kansas vs. Marks* (1982), the court found that "rape trauma syndrome was relevant to the issue of whether a woman consented to sexual intercourse." The police have developed more compassionate ways of dealing with rape victims, including first contacts by female officers who are trained to provide more sensitive and less threatening interrogations.

Rape no longer has the terrible stigma it once had in years past. Women no longer must feel their "shame" in secret. Today's outreach programs, crisis centers, support groups, and prevention classes help soften the terrible impact of rape, including its inevitable aftershock.

PRESSURE POINT FIVE: MURDER ONE

Statistics show that most of the murders committed in this country are crimes of passion, executed by people who knew the victim and were either welcomed into his or her house or were already living under the same roof. This shock of betrayal adds a paralyzing element to an already traumatic event.

Even surviving an attempted murder can bring a rash of aftershock symptoms along with relief—from agoraphobia, fear of public places, to paranoia. This was carried to the ultimate in Jules Feiffer's film *Little Murders*, where the city became a suspicion-built prison, with everyone trying to kill everyone else.

Aftershock can also entrap people who knew and loved a victim of murder. These innocent sufferers can become obsessed with revenge and take justice into their own hands.

And thanks to newspaper coverage, publicity campaigns, and media blitzes in today's information age, aftershock can turn up in people who never even knew the murder victim. Fifteen years ago, there was a psychopath on the loose in New York City, who called himself "The Son of Sam." This unknown assailant stalked the city streets, killing young girls with long hair. Until the police found him, after a dramatic manhunt, young girls all over the city could be seen riding the subways to work with their hair up or wearing scarves, living in fear that it would happen to them. They so strongly identified with the girls that were killed that they too suffered severe anxiety.

PRESSURE POINT SIX: THE MASKED BANDITS

Robbery and assault: Twin crimes with far-reaching repercussions. In 1986 alone, over 540,000 Americans were robbed and over 830,000 were victims of aggravated assault (figures derived from the Federal Bureau of Investigation, *Crime in the United States*). Chances are you know somebody who has been burglarized or attacked. Perhaps you have been a victim yourself, feeling a sense of violation at the thought of an anonymous person creeping through your belongings. Afterward when the trauma has passed, people will put in elaborate alarm systems as a way of controlling their fear and of regaining a sense of power over a situation that took them by surprise. The facts bear this out. Alarm system installers get most of their orders from people who have already been robbed.

Assault victims also learn wisdom after the fall. Maybe they don't go out at night; perhaps they begin to avoid crime-heavy areas. Some may buy and register guns and carry them with them.

Both robbery and assault share in producing loss of innocence. Whether you read about a robbery in the papers or fall prey to a mugging, you can no longer go out without looking over your shoulder, without making sure your car is locked, without feeling distrustful of strangers. This "street-smart" aftershock behavior, rare in past generations, evidences a pressure point that is a real disease of our times.

COMMUNITY DISASTERS

They might be God's will, but these events cause tremendous aftershock in their wake. From earthquakes, tornadoes, floods, and fires to the man-made disasters of our nuclear age, all can inflict aftershock on a vast scale.

PRESSURE POINT SEVEN: ACTS OF GOD

Blood, frogs, pestilence, locusts, darkness—the plagues that befell Ancient Egypt were truly acts of God. Today's world has its own brand of plagues.

One of the most documented community disasters was the one that took place at Buffalo Creek, West Virginia in 1972. It had been raining hard throughout the state. The Buffalo Creek dam kept the water at bay until it was undermined through a fault in its structure. A raging torrent flooded the entire town—sudden, violent, and deadly. Eighty percent of the survivors succumbed to aftershock, and five years later 30 percent still had as severe a case as they had had at the outset. Only one out of every five citizens of Buffalo Creek had *no* symptoms of aftershock.

Why so violent a reaction? Part of the reason was its sudden, uncontrollable, and unavoidable nature. But there was more to it than that. Though it was a flood, an act of God, that caused the swollen dam, it was the *man-made* dam that broke and brought the flood to town. If the dam had been structurally sound, the flood would never have occurred.

In the minds of the citizens of Buffalo Creek there was always the thought that it didn't have to happen. No one can stop an act of God, but a man-made dam could have been built better. Someone along the way could have prevented the tragedy. Added to the trauma of death and devastation, the people felt anger—at the dam's developers, at the government, at themselves. The crisis intensified; the aftershock symptoms snowballed, moving from spouse to spouse, child to child, neighborhood to neighborhood. After the event,

- 30 percent increased their alcohol consumption,
- 44 percent increased their cigarette smoking,
- 52 percent started taking prescription drugs,
- 12 percent became juvenile delinquents, and two years later,
- 75 percent more people suffered from insomnia!

Proof positive that community disaster and aftershock go hand in hand. The following examples provide more evidence.

- Twenty out of the fifty firemen in South Australia who got caught up in a huge 1983 bushfire developed PTSD, and only one sought help. Four years later, twelve firemen still displayed aftershock symptoms, including intruding, debilitating memories and lapses in concentration.
- Eighty-seven out of ninety-nine victims of the Mt. St. Helens eruption had at least one episode of PTSD.
- A raging fire in a crowded restaurant caused the 1942 Coconut Grove disaster in Boston. The Holy Cross football team had just won an important game over Boston College. Over 500 men, women, and children were out celebrating the victory (or sharing the sorrow of defeat); most were in festive spirits, eating, drinking, and cheering, when the fire broke out. Fire exits were blocked and panic quickly set in. Four hundred and ninety-one died, and

aftershock had a holiday. One father kept dreaming about the daughter he lost in the fire, dreaming that she was in a telephone booth calling him for help. A man who lost his wife seemed fine when he left the hospital after treatment for his minor scraps and burns. But a few days later, he returned. He was on edge and he had morbid thoughts. He kept saying over and over, "I should have saved her or I should have died too." He was admitted back into the hospital, and on the sixth day of his hospital stay he jumped out of a window to his death. A young teenage girl lost her entire family in the fire. But she seemed to be handling her trauma fairly well. She discussed her feelings with the doctors and was cheerful toward the nurses and other patients. There was no reason to keep her in the hospital and she was released. Her uncontrollable crying didn't start until she had been home a week. Soon she was weeping nonstop. She was unable to function. Only treatment would help her lead a normal life.

A lack of control is inherent in a natural disaster. We can learn how to read the signs before an earthquake or a hurricane begins, but we cannot stop the earth's tremors or the sky's torrential downpours. We can only learn to reduce nature's damage—and reduce our risk of aftershock. The four questions that can make all the difference between developing PTSD or coming out unscathed are

1. Was your life in danger and if so for how long?

2. Did many people die, and were there among them people you loved?

3. Were you exposed to the trauma for a long period of time?

4. How well organized were the social services and rescue teams after the natural disaster occurred?

PRESSURE POINT EIGHT: MAN-MADE WASTE

Guilt—it's what separates the implications of a natural disaster from those of man-made waste. Since you can't prevent an act of God, you don't have to suffer any guilt. (Though people do feel the ramifications of surviving when others have not.) But a man-made disaster might have been stopped—if you had seen it coming; if you had the defect fixed; if, like the little Dutch boy of nursery rhyme fame, you had plugged up the leak all by yourself. In a study following the Mt. St. Helens disaster it was discovered that only 42 percent of the aftershock victims suffered from guilt, as opposed to 80 percent of the interviewed women who had been victims of rape.

Man-made disasters are insidious. It's as if technology, the hope of the future, suddenly revealed itself a beast that took the helm in a bizarre science-fiction adventure: "Mad machines go haywire! Creators slaughtered!" But toxic fallouts are very real, and they are not funny. Three-Mile Island and more recently Chernobyl have brought the downside of our advanced technological state into fierce focus.

Adding fuel to the man-made fire is the fact that toxic afteraffects can take years to develop. A tornado hits then moves on. Technological disasters look invisible at first; they unfold slowly. It took a week before the Three-Mile Island leak was discovered, and today many neighboring citizens are still worried about radiation damage.

The invisible nature of certain dangers creates a passivity in people. Take for example the radon hazard in Upper Montclair, New Jersey. A harmful gas, invisible and odorless, produced naturally from decaying elements below the earth's surface, radon was discovered in

---

CHERNOBYL: THEN AND NOW

April 1986. Chernobyl becomes the byword for nuclear reactor disasters as it releases the largest amount of radioactivity ever recorded during a single technological accident. But is the Chernobyl incident a hideous *China Syndrome* come true? Two years later, the facts remain unclear. Some experts say Chernobyl will ultimately cause between 20,000 and 40,000 cancer-related deaths. Others claim the total figure will be less—only .02% of all cancer deaths.

Because of Chernobyl, governments have enacted new laws and regulations regarding food control, safety measures, radiation monitoring, emergency procedures, and emergency management. To be forewarned is to be forearmed. Maybe . . .

dangerous concentrations in several homes. The government offered free radon check tests for other homeowners. There was very little response. People couldn't see the radon; they couldn't smell it or taste it. Just as San Franciscans avert their thoughts from the possibility of earthquakes, and German Jews refused for too long to heed the danger from Hitler, homeowners refused to think their homes, their havens, were potentially lethal.

The situation was totally different when the government wanted to dump fairly low-grade radioactive refuse in Vernon, New Jersey. Here, citizens were up in arms; there was a flurry of protest. Why the difference? Because this time people had someone to blame and not just anybody—the distrusted government. And because this time the people had a physical object, radioactive waste, to protest against, not just the invisible poison of radon gas.

Another fallout from man-made waste is its constant replaying. Stress stays alive when lawsuits, protests, and media coverage keep it fresh. It's hard to put the past to rest when you are actively involved in the story.

CURRENT EVENTS

You only have to look at today's headlines to feel the almost routine shock of daily life worldwide. Current events have their own global impact, their own potency, their own aftershock value.

PRESSURE POINT NINE: LEADER ASSASSINATION

The privilege of power also has its dangers, especially that deadly symbol of protest: assassination. From Alexander the Great to Ronald Reagan, leaders have always needed bodyguards to ward off the death threats, the psychotic, delusional protestors, the murderous weapons of the misguided. But it was not until John F. Kennedy was shot and the event shown on national TV that most Americans felt assassination's aftershock. Suddenly, we were no longer invincible. Suddenly, we knew the political terrorism that had always afflicted other countries. How many of us remember, twenty-odd years later, where we were and what we were doing when JFK was shot? How many of us remember watching Bobby Kennedy's funeral train on television, sobbing out of control as our eyes stayed glued to the set? Or feeling the dead weight of hopelessness when Martin Luther King was killed? Assassins' bullets hit our leaders and we get the fallout.

PRESSURE POINT TEN: MISSING!

When did our friendly milk cartons become bedecked with the faces of kidnapped children? When did we stop letting our kids go out to play alone? When did bizarre behavior become the norm, forcing us to fear the worst? Unfortunately, kidnapping has become a common fear for American families.

PRESSURE POINT ELEVEN: TAKEN HOSTAGE!

In 1976, twenty-six children ranging from five to fourteen, were taken hostage in Chowchilla, California. They were buried alive in their school bus for twenty-seven hours before they dug themselves out. All twenty six developed PTSD. In 1983, the twenty-six children were interviewed, and though their aftershock symptoms were less severe, they still

/ Reenacted the trauma when they played
/ Had difficulty understanding the time and place of the trauma
/ Felt a hopelessness about their future

The darkness of hostage-taking has one ray of light; it unites a country. When the hostages were taken in Iran, Americans came together in a common cause—to get them out. We counted off the days along with our newscasters. We tied yellow ribbons on our trees. We prayed and cried along with the hostages' families. And as some political analysts suggested, we cheered the hostages' homecoming more than we ever had that of our returning Vietnam vets.

PRESSURE POINT TWELVE: THE GROWING HOMELESS!

"There but for the grace of God go I." They are seen sleeping in our train stations, huddling on street corners, crowding into makeshift shelters. They are the homeless—and their numbers are growing. Billy Boggs might have championed her right to live on the streets if she so chose, but most of our homeless want a way back if they haven't completely given up in despair. Though there are many alcoholic or mentally unstable people out on the streets, the majority got merely through a stunning string of bad luck. Maybe they lost their jobs and couldn't pay their mortgages or rents. Maybe they had no family and nowhere to turn. Maybe they became ill and couldn't work up the strength to keep going. Whatever the reason, today they have no home for themselves or for their children. Listen:

In 1980 1,400 children lived in welfare hotels. By 1987 the figure rose to 12,000. In *USA Today* Dr. Irwin Redlener, who worked in a mobile unit at the various hotels, likened these children to Ethiopian famine victims. They are not immunized. They are neglected. They are missing the basic children's health care we have come to expect in our society. He has seen them come in with everything from heart murmurs and dehydration to asthma and ear infections.

The sight and plight of the homeless affects us to the core. We feel both guilt and despair at a problem that only gets bigger—with no end in sight.

PRESSURE POINT THIRTEEN: PLANE CRASH!

How many of us have been afraid to fly after hearing about a recent plane crash? How many of us must drink ourselves practically unconscious before we can handle a takeoff without fear? We are not alone. The next time you are in an airport note how close the bars are to the gates, and note how many people are trying vainly to relieve their anxiety.

Anxiety over flying makes sense. For one hour, four hours, even ten hours, we must relinquish control to an anonymous pilot as we fly thousands of miles thousands of feet above the earth. Even though we are told that more people die in car crashes every year than in airplanes, we close our ears. After all, we have control of the car; our hands are on the wheel. Not so with planes.

As a doctor I have seen dead bodies in hospital wards and corridors since the first day I entered med school. Though one never gets used to the sight, they come with the territory. But if I saw a dead body on a lovely country landscape, I would feel completely different. Dead bodies belong in morgues, not on sun-filled meadows. For care-givers and rescuers rushed to the crash scene, this "out of context" element

---

SURVIVAL

On October 12, 1972, a Fairchild F227 took off from Montevideo, Uruguay, bound for Santiago, Chile. Inside were fifteen members of an amateur rugby team and twenty-five of their family and friends plus a small crew. Because of stormy weather, the plane stopped overnight in the small town of Mendoza, in Argentina. It took off again the next day . . . and crashed into the Andes mountains at 3:30 p.m.

At first, thirty-two survivors of the crash tried to stay alive in the plane's shattered fuselage, subsisting on wine and bits of candy. The numbers kept dropping. By the time a Chilean peasant spied a bedraggled, emaciated survivor ten weeks later, only sixteen remained.

The survivors gained notoriety because they had resorted to cannibalism to stay alive. But their story is more than sensationalism. It is a testament to the determination of the human spirit to stay alive—and remain sane.

---

adds even more stress to the traumatic event, and it helps them develop aftershock.

When a Pacific Southwest Airline commuter plane went down in San Luis County, California in 1987, psychologists were brought to the scene to help the rescuers deal with the sight of forty-three bodies, many of them mutilated. Even hardened emergency-room doctors and nurses need help in dealing with this kind of crisis. As the head of the San Luis Obispo Mental Health Department told *USA Today*, "I don't think human beings are wired to deal with that kind of trauma."

According to Dr. Stephen Xenakis, care-givers, police officers, and firemen can avoid aftershock on the job with:

- Strong leadership
- Clear delineation of duties
- Time on the scene to mourn the loss
- An organized plan of mental health services—for both long-term and short-term therapy

PRESSURE POINT FOURTEEN: NUCLEAR THREAT!

Madonna might sing about the material world, but teenagers today call it a nuclear world. They are growing up under a mushroom cloud that is much deadlier than previous generations believed. They know that crawling under a desk during an air-raid drill or building fallout shelters in the basement can't stop nuclear winter. Radiation ultimately kills. Period.

In *Psychiatry '87*, antinuclear activist Dr. Eric Chivian interviewed both Soviet and American children and discovered a wide discrepancy in their views. Fifty percent of the Soviet children believed nuclear war would never happen. But only 14 percent of the 3,300 American high school students he interviewed were as optimistic. An overwhelming 42 percent believed there would someday be a nuclear war.

Are American teenagers more pessimistic? Not really. It's just that our youths have grown up with movies like *The Terminator* and *Road Warrior*, and with TV specials like *The Day After*, all with storylines that emphasize the possibility, even the likelihood of nuclear war.

PRESSURE POINT FIFTEEN: THE AIDS SCARE!

No one today is untouched by this once obscure virus. It has caused shock waves throughout our world and has irrevocably changed the way we view sex and love.

AIDS cuts at our primal urge for intimacy. No longer can we get solace in another person's arms without at least thinking of a thorough blood test. Many young adults are staying virgins. Others worry that their next sexual encounter may be their last.

AIDS patients have come into hospitals with rotting teeth because they could not get a dentist to work on them. They come in with false names. They spend thousands of dollars on health care because they won't use their office's insurance plan for fear of discovery. They are ostracized if they don't keep their disease a secret. And they are robbed of emotional support from family and friends if they do.

AIDS has been compared to leprosy. Both have been of epidemic proportions. Both have made their victims outcasts. Both have built up an irrational fear. But the lessons from the past can stop AIDS from controlling our lives. Before we mistakenly begin carting its victims off to isolated islands, we must look inside ourselves. We must realize that just as those who succumbed to leprosy did nothing wrong, so is it true with AIDS victims. Read on:

✎ A family whose three children had AIDS only wanted their children to go to school and lead a somewhat normal life. Their house was burned to the ground.

✎ A Massachusetts family is slowly being wiped out because the mother received a tainted blood transfusion when she gave birth to her first child. She went on to have two more children without knowing she had developed AIDS. Her husband has been recently diagnosed as AIDS positive. Only one four-year-old daughter is free of the disease.

✎ A young and talented artist has only one homosexual lover and still comes down with AIDS.

There is no blame here; only a disease that is out of control. Tremendous progress has already been made, and someday soon there will be a cure. In the meantime, as Dr. Douglas Shenson writes in *The New York Times Magazine*, "The point is not to be scared, but to be careful. The greatest occupational hazard in caring for my patients is not in catching the disease, but rather in falling victim to the emotional brutalization that comes with the work."

What we have are people—ordinary people who need, if not our help, at least our understanding.

The problems of today, the prophecies of tomorrow: They overcome us, yet we cannot let them stop us. We must make good choices. We must live life to the best of our abilities.

To everything there is a season. Let us pray for spring.

We have just looked at the worldwide trauma-causing events of the 1980s, the impersonal events that hit home. In the next chapter we will go on to "crimes of the heart" and examine the traumas that occur one-on-one and that affect us in a deep, personal way.

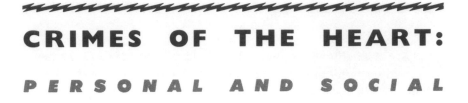

CRIMES OF THE HEART:

PERSONAL AND SOCIAL

8

Menschen, menschen, san ma all . . .
(Human, human are we all . . .)
A VIENNESE SAYING

HUMANITY IS A STUDY IN CONTRASTS. ON ONE hand, we have no desire to know what is in store down the road, especially if the news is bad. On the other hand, we check out our horoscope daily. We seek out fortune tellers and crystal gazers. We want to know—and we don't.

But even a psychic knows there are no guarantees. Change — sometimes sudden, sometimes gradual—is the one certainty of life. A loved one can die. You can fall in love and marry. A friend can get sick. You can inherit a great deal of money, changing your life drastically.

As the song goes, "Something's lost, but something's gained, in living every day." But these things, both the losses and the gains, can throw us a curve. Like a fast ball thrown too fast they can knock the wind out of us, leaving us to find aftershock in the dust.

THE SCALES OF STRESS

Each of the life-changing events below happen to people every day. Before I go on to today's personal pressure points, take a moment to look them over. Created by Drs. Thomas Holmes and Richard Rahe, this test is designed to help you see how much stress you are experiencing right now. Check off any crisis that you have had within the past twelve months, putting the number of times you have experienced the event in the "mean value" column. Multiply that number by the number you see next to the event. Put the total in the "stress index" column. Count up your total "stress index" figures and you will have the amount of stress you may be feeling. Below 150 means your life should be coasting along just fine. From 150 to 199 you might be experiencing some mild stress. A total from 200 to 299 suggests that this is a time of moderate stress for you. And a score above 300 points to major stress and could very well mean you are in the throes of serious aftershock.

You will notice that these positive and negative life events are almost all unavoidable. Unless you spend your life in a box, you will experience many of these traumas as you continue to grow. Living holds a certain amount of stress. Learning to handle this stress will make your life a healthier and happier one, and recognizing the pressure points that will arise can help you avoid the more serious repercussions of aftershock. Let's go over the main personal and social pressure points right now.

RITES OF PASSAGE

Other rituals, other times. In primitive tribes, a young boy on the brink of adulthood must walk through fire and paint his face to prove he is a man. In nineteenth-century England a gentleman proved his mettle by the way he knotted his tie. In the court of Louis XIV a woman proclaimed her marital status by the way she wore a beauty mark on her cheek.

Our customs would probably look as equally strange to a traveler from 2401. But if the rituals change, the reasons behind them are timeless; they are a part of the natural cycles of life, marked by marriage, death, birth, divorce. Whether these events call for celebration or mourning, they are very real, very basic, and they come with their own pressure point stress.

Life Event in the
Last Twelve Months

Life Event in the Last Twelve Months	Mean Value	Stress Index
Death of spouse	____ × 100	____
Divorce	____ × 73	____
Marital separation	____ × 65	____
Jail term	____ × 63	____
Death of close family member	____ × 63	____
Personal injury or illness	____ × 53	____
Marriage	____ × 50	____
Fired at work	____ × 47	____
Marital reconciliation	____ × 45	____
Retirement	____ × 45	____
Change in health of family member(s)	____ × 44	____
Pregnancy	____ × 40	____
Sex difficulties	____ × 39	____
Gain of new family member	____ × 39	____
Business readjustment	____ × 39	____
Change in financial state	____ × 38	____

Death of close friend	____ × 37	____
Change of careers	____ × 36	____
Change in number of arguments with spouse	____ × 35	____
Mortgage over $10,000	____ × 31	____
Foreclosure of mortgage or loan	____ × 30	____
Change in work responsibilities	____ × 29	____
Son or daughter leaving home	____ × 29	____
In-law trouble	____ × 29	____
Outstanding personal achievement	____ × 28	____
Spouse beginning or stopping work	____ × 26	____
Beginning or ending school	____ × 26	____
Change in living conditions	____ × 25	____
Revision of personal habits	____ × 24	____
Boss trouble	____ × 23	____
Change in work conditions and hours	____ × 20	____
Change in residence	____ × 20	____

Change in schools	_____ ×	20	_____
Change in recreation	_____ ×	19	_____
Change in religious activities	_____ ×	19	_____
Change in social activities	_____ ×	18	_____
Mortgage or loan less than $10,000	_____ ×	17	_____
Change in sleeping habits	_____ ×	16	_____
Change in number of family get-togethers	_____ ×	15	_____
Change in eating habits	_____ ×	15	_____
Vacation	_____ ×	13	_____
Christmas	_____ ×	12	_____
Minor violations of the law	_____ ×	11	_____
	TOTAL =		_____

Reprinted with permission from *American Health* magazine.

Ironically, as common to all as these rites of passage are, they are also the most unique. Your marriage is different from any other marriage. You experience the death of a loved one in a different way from anyone else. The way you love your new baby is so unique you cannot express it in words.

PRESSURE POINT SIXTEEN: LOVE AND MARRIAGE

In centuries past, the bride occasionally wore black. And love had nothing to do with it. Marriages were arranged way in advance, usually when a man and woman were just children living miles apart. It was as political as war, a way of uniting countries and fortunes, of uplifting one's social standing. Today's world is different. People are marrying for love—or what they hope will be love. With both partners working, financial needs are no longer the consideration they once were. Executive women are marrying carpenters. Men are becoming house husbands and housewives are entering the work-force en masse. Compassion, sensitivity, and support have become the ideals in a prospective spouse. But this ability to look for more emotional fulfillment is balanced with cynicism. How many times have you heard: "She's a great first wife" or "Oh, this is my first marriage" or "I need a wedding present that can be split up—just in case"?

With divorce and extramarital affairs as commonplace as VCRs, it's easy to see why these attitudes prevail. But hope springs eternal. And in actuality the percentage of marriages in this country is as high as the divorce rate.

In a world with so many options, so many choices, marriage is a stressful proposition, When you get married, you flout the odds and say "I love you till death do us part." You are saying that you are prepared to share the rest of your life with one person—no matter what vicisitudes you both will have to face. It's a turning point in the most dramatic sense.

In a study of six couples embarking on marriage, Dr. Rhona Rapoport found that the best results for happiness came if both husband and wife are

Ⅰ **Realistically ready to take on their new, more dependent role as a couple—including a willingness to share a home, financial responsibility, and planning for the future**

2   Ready to change relationships that would interfere with their newly formed commitment and dependency, such as the tie to a child who is accustomed to close involvement with the formerly single parent, colleagues who keep suggesting drinks after work, and friends who continue to call late at night

3   Able to confront their differences and accept compromise—be it that the husband hates to dance and the wife can't imagine life without a dance floor, or that the husband craves freedom and the wife clings to him night and day.

But opposites *do* attract, and a couple with different interests and values can have a good fit. A case in point: a woman who loves her corporate life and a laid back man can become better people together, complementing each other's role and giving each other a different viewpoint, a "reality check" on the world outside their respective spheres.

On the other hand, two people with similar interests might not get along together at all. If that same executive woman married an equally high-powered executive man, they both might find that their needs are not being met, that each one has no time to spare to nurture the other.

Love might be lovelier the second time around, but the stress is no less severe. On the plus side, people in second marriages have more experience in the world of relationships. Hopefully, their first marriage has taught them to read the warning signs before divorce once more rears its ugly head. They have a clearer picture of what they need and what they want from a relationship than couples walking down the aisle for the first time. And as couples in second marriages are usually older, they are more independent and more willing to join in an interdependent relationship.

On the minus side, there is a tremendous anxiety that this marriage too will not work. To fail twice is much more difficult to accept than to fail only once. There is an old adage, "Once shame on you, twice shame on me." If a person hasn't worked out the problems of the past or has married someone exactly like this or her ex-spouse, there is always the very real possibility of another failure.

What about planning the marriage itself? That too creates its own pressure point. Take the case of Amy, a young woman who wanted to get married above anything else. She loved John, her husband to be, but he was almost an abstraction to her, the crucial piece for her white dress, church wedding, and Caribbean honeymoon. For over a year, she planned her wedding, taking time off from work to interview bands, florists, and photographers, spending her weekends searching high and low for the perfect dress.

Yes, the wedding turned out to be beautiful. The bride was in her glory; everyone had a wonderful time. But five hours later it was over. In another week, the honeymoon was only a memory. Several months later, a friend saw Amy at another wedding. They chatted; Amy couldn't stop talking about *her* wedding. She had lived for the moment, without thinking about the realities of married life: the finances, the daily routines, the intense sharing. Ultimately, Amy worked out her problems with her husband. But she had learned a difficult lesson; the goal of marriage is not marriage itself. It's two people sharing a life, sharing a heart, in turbulent, troubled times. It is caring, nurturing, and communicating—long after the dizzy weeks of early romance.

PRESSURE POINT SEVENTEEN: DIVORCE

No one who enters a marriage really believes he or she will get a divorce. Even those who take a hard-headed approach, with prenuptial contracts, will always feel, if and when the time comes, that emotional element that defies logic: the fact that their marriage is headed for divorce—and will be hurt.

According to columnist Jane Brody divorce "can exact a greater and in many cases longer-lasting emotional and physical toll on the former spouses than virtually any other life stress, including widowhood."

Divorced couples have higher rates of

- Suicide and alcoholism
- Heart disease and cancer
- Accidents and emotional problems
- High blood pressure and pneumonia

In fact, the emotional and physical problems that divorced people have are usually a direct result of the broken marriage, and not symptoms of an earlier and previously undetected illness. Even among smokers, divorced men showed a higher rate of death than their married, cigarette-addicted counterparts.

Like the death of a loved one, divorce holds much grief, depression, and anger—with one crucial extra element; the ex-spouse is still alive. It is more difficult for a divorced person to go through the normal process of grief because there is continued contact, even if it's just in a chance remark from a mutual friend.

The aftershock symptoms of divorce usually last about three years, though custody battles, financial pressures, and continued contact can make them last even longer. There have been cases of sexual dysfunction years after the divorce and even after a man or woman had happily remarried. A study of men and women who were separated or divorced and who had sought psychiatric help, found that they did not improve over a fourteen-month period following their breakup, and in many cases their problems got worse. The study also found that women are more emotionally wrung out *before* the separation, while men suffer much more *after* the breakup has taken place.

The spouses who initiate the divorce might be in for harder times than the spouses who hear the news. They have to suffer with the guilt that they are causing pain to someone who has shared their life. They have made the difficult decision to leave the comfort and security of the known to face an uncertain future, an "aggressive" stance that keeps needed sympathy and support from others at bay. Further, there is the fact that they feel ready for divorce; they are prepared and excited about the prospect of beginning anew as a "free" man or woman. But life is never what one envisions, and many initiators find, six months down the road, that they are disappointed in their freedom. More times than not, they will ultimately ask for a reconciliation.

The surprised victims, on the other hand, are initially filled with pain and terror. Even if they had seen the signs that the marriage was dissolving, they denied them. As a Spanish philosopher once said: "It's better to sit at the table with a known devil than court a strange angel." But because they had no exciting, preconceived notions of what life would be like alone—and indeed were terrified of the prospect of such a life—they feel much less disappointment than their ex-spouses. Bolstered with the sympathy and support that, because of their victim role, is more freely given, they find themselves pleasantly surprised. After several months, life begins to look up, and if the initiators suggest a reconciliation, more times than not, the victims say no.

For a smoother, less stressful divorce:

⚡ Keep communication with your ex-spouse to a minimum, even if children are involved.

⚡ Involve yourself with a support group or a circle of friends. A good support system is vital to keeping your spirits up.

⚡ Whenever your spirits flag, remind yourself that as miserable as you might feel, studies show that people who stay together in an unhappy marriage are more anxious and depressed than divorced couples.

⚡ Though there is a real tendency to take up with old friends who have shut out your ex-spouse, it's best to avoid them. Studies prove they cause more emotional stress than friends who have kept a relationship going with the both of you.

⚡ Don't use courtroom battles to seek revenge, with appeal after appeal to get your just deserts. Fights will only continue to keep the trauma alive and stop you from going forward in your life.

⚡ Be open to new relationships. They can help you recover faster from the trauma of divorce.

⚡ Don't hesitate to seek help if you are feeling overwhelmed. Therapy can stop debilitating aftershock symptoms from cropping up.

The good news is that 75 percent of all divorced women and 80 percent of all divorced men fall in love again and marry.

PRESSURE POINT EIGHTEEN: BIRTH

Congratulations! You are having a baby. It's exciting, it's exhilarating, it's terrifying. Even as you are setting up the nursery and planning a future, you are worried about your baby's health, about finances, about your life completely changing. These feelings are very real, very normal —and very stressful.

One episode of the TV series *St. Elsewhere* showed Dr. Ehrlich and his pregnant wife, Lucy, talking in bed about their baby-to-be. Their discussion began very romantically. He talked of his little boy, his hopes, and dreams. She smiled contentedly, thinking of her new-born in her arms. Suddenly, there was a reality shift as they got into finances. They spoke of the cost of living, of college tuition, of the responsibilities involved. It was a fearful proposition. They stopped talking. Fiction, yes, but it mirrors real life. As much as we prepare for a new baby, we cannot truly experience parenting until we bring our newborn home. We can only do our best and hope our child will grow up healthy and happy. To paraphrase the famous Dr. Spock: "Trust your instincts. Chances are you will be right."

When the joys of birth are doubled, they also bring double trouble. With twins, the cost of raising baby suddenly jumps twofold: two cribs, two carriages, two packages of diapers, two sets of clothes. And in today's world twins are more common than you think—there are over 2.4 million sets of twins in the United States and an estimated 33,000 sets of twins are born each year.

Why this increase in twin births? Possibly because mothers are taking better care of themselves than ever before. Possibly because many women are waiting until they are older to have children. And possibly because these older mothers-to-be are taking fertility medication. Whichever the case, the best antidote to the trauma of twins is information. Many books are currently being published about raising twins, answering questions on every issue from breastfeeding to establishing synchronized nap times.

Whether a single newborn or a set of twins, birth is stressful to new parents. But it cannot come close to the pain of *not* giving birth, of miscarrying your baby-to-be. Mothers who miscarry have been known to walk around depressed and anxious long after the event. Many mothers cannot find the strength to pack up the nursery or get on with life. The slightest stimulus, a babyfood commercial or a baby carriage passing on the street, can set them off. In fact, to help prevent this tragedy, the Jewish religion does not allow baby showers until after the baby is born. In addition to the superstitious motive, a desire not to tempt the fates, it also has a practical purpose: If a mother miscarries, there won't be any cribs or baby furniture to remind her of the pain.

Sometimes a miscarriage can trigger a trauma from the past. A case in point is a woman who had survived several years in a concentration camp. She emigrated to America, married, and became pregnant. When she miscarried, her depression was much worse than might have been expected. Her loss reminded her of that awful time when she had seen children led to the gas chamber.

Premature birth holds much the same pain as miscarriage, at least until the baby is out of danger. David Kaplan and Edward Masan at The Harvard School of Public Health, Family Guidance Center studied sixty families who recently went through the trauma of a premature birth. Here's what the Center found:

FULL-TERM PREGNANCY:	PREMATURE BIRTH:
A woman comes into the hospital with the belief she is doing something healthy and normal.	A woman is brought in on an emergency basis. She feels the fear of crisis.
Mother-to-be can be given an anesthetic.	Mother-to-be must deliver without medication for fear the child can be harmed.
New mother receives congratulations on a happy job well done. Receives support from doctors and others.	Mother-to-be must recuperate from ordeal. Suffers anxiety over baby's well-being. No congratulations, only suspense.
Anxiety eases as mother takes care of her new baby's normal needs.	Anxiety heightened in life-and-death situation.
Mother put in ward with other happy new moms.	Mother put in ward where some of the women have lost their babies.
Nursery filled with happy, healthy babies.	Nursery on other floor; tiny baby consumed by oxygen tanks and tubes.

FULL-TERM PREGNANCY:·	PREMATURE BIRTH:
Mother returns home with baby, ready to assume new role.	Mother returns home empty-handed and depressed.
Mother learns to care for normal baby via instinct and support.	When baby comes home, there is more anxiety over weight gain and illness.

As stressful as a premature birth is, there are ways to remedy the situation and cushion the blows of aftershock. The mother-to-be should be prepared for possible death with "anticipatory grief." But as her baby improves, so must her hope. Yes, there are extra responsibilities to deal with at home, but they are only temporary. As the baby continues to grow, so will the new mother's confidence.

PRESSURE POINT NINETEEN: DEATH OF A LOVED ONE

Passed away—gone—no more. No matter what we call it, death hurts. The grief, that yawning absence of someone you love, is inexplicably painful. The loss can never be forgotten, only accepted and assimilated into a new view of life without that person. People can continue mourning for years, without even realizing it. When they seek help, it's usually not for the loss they suffered. It is only later, after therapy has begun, that the truth of death's aftershock comes out.

In normal grief, a person will go through six stages of acceptance similar to the Kübler-Ross stages I talked about in Chapter Four. Specifically, a mourner's immediate reaction will be to do something for the deceased, usually a funeral they would have liked, because the full impact of the death has yet to strike. Next a mourner will deny the death, ignoring the feelings of pain and sadness, though he or she might dream vividly about the deceased. (If people get stuck in this stage, they may begin to abuse alcohol or drugs or work themselves up into a sexual, exercise, or business frenzy.) Once past this denial stage, a mourner begins to review his or her life with the dead: memories are vivid and emotions are high. Finally, in a last-ditch attempt to deny the loss, a mourner will feel a tremendous yearning for the deceased, which in turn leads to acceptance and the ability to enjoy life once more.

The pain of surviving, that overwhelming sense of loss, sadness, and even anger at the dead, stops after six or nine months. But it's not unusual for people to grieve for one or two years longer, especially if it is a spouse who had died suddenly.

Unfinished mourning and acute grief reactions are a part of aftershock's siren call. Whether it has been six months or ten years after a loved one had died, these symptoms live on:

↯ **A numb, flat feeling**

↯ **A resistance in finishing projects or meeting new people**

↯ **A need to keep a memento of the deceased around all the time. (One woman kept her dead husband's keys hanging in her kitchen window so she would think of him whenever she saw the keys.)**

↯ **A tendency to sigh frequently, combined with a tightness in the throat**

↯ **A complete lack of energy**

↯ **An empty feeling in one's stomach even after eating**

↯ **A preoccupation with the dead loved one, as if the deceased were still around (One man who lost a close friend in a terrible fire talked to the deceased over the dinner table.)**

↯ **A tremendously guilty feeling, no matter how irrational, that one was responsible for the death**

↯ **Anger and coldness toward others, especially to family and friends who are trying to give support and sympathy**

↯ **A lack of focus and an automatic way of dealing with daily routines**

↯ **An inability to carry on a normal conversation**

↯ **A taking on of the deceased's behavior, as if the dead person had entered one's body (One woman began to use her hands the way her father had. She saw him in the mirror instead of herself. She actually changed careers to pursue goals that her father would have liked.)**

Aftershock happens more often if the mourner had been ambivalent about the deceased, if there had been some anger and guilt expressed right before the death. Take Chris. He had gone to visit his father a week before his father's death. They had had a terrific fight about Chris's career. His father wanted him to enter the family business; Chris wanted to get a Ph.D. in philosophy. They had bitter words and Chris hadn't called his father all week. On Sunday night of the second week, Chris went to sleep, only to have the phone wake him up at 4:00 a.m. His father had had a massive heart attack and he was dead. Chris had a double whammy. Not only did he begin to feel guilty about the fight he had had with his father but the suddenness of his father's death added to the shock.

When someone dies after a long bout of illness, there is more time to prepare, though, as I discussed in Chapter Three, a sense of unfairness is still present in the trauma. But as long as the time together is not used to deny the approaching death, it's a real opportunity to set grievances straight, to rehash old problems, and to bring harmony into each other's lives.

A religious belief always helps in the face of death; it provides a strength and a meaning to the loss. The rituals soothe and comfort; they take the mourners' minds off their suffering, and they help stall the grieving process until the shock of the trauma can be better handled. Think of the Irish wake or the Jewish shiva, where friends and families crowd together to share food, drink, and solace. Memories and tears are exchanged; the reality that life goes on is reinforced.

But in the tragic death of a child, even rituals can barely help. A child is a part of the future and, for the surviving parents, there will always be that unfulfilled, unanswered promise in their lives. As Dr. George Pollack told the *New York Times*, "Mourning is never completed."

A poignant note comes from coach Bob Wagner, who taught Len Bias at Northwestern High School before Len became the University of Maryland's basketball star—and before he died of a drug overdose. After Len's death, Wagner quit his job and became a hermit. He didn't answer the phone. He didn't eat for days at a time. He was completely wrenched. As Wagner told *USA Today*, "I was accepting responsibility for what had happened to Lenny, blaming myself. I kept thinking, 'What didn't I do right? What should I have taught that I hadn't?' "

The coach ultimately got over his pain and went back to coaching. He accepted the death and realized it was not his fault or his responsibility that Len Bias died.

Death is difficult for anyone to handle. We never know how we will react. It is our worst fear confirmed; we really are not going to live forever.

PRESSURE POINT TWENTY: SUICIDE

Death at any time is difficult to accept, but to actively seek it out is devastating. Suicide is the ultimate selfish deed. As Woody Allen's character in _Hannah and Her Sisters_ said, "I was going to kill myself. The only thing that mighta stopped me, might've, is my parents would be devastated. I would, I woulda had to shoot them also, first. And then, I have an aunt and uncle, I would have. . . . You know, it would have been a bloodbath."

Part of grief's healing process involves talk. But families and friends of a suicide victim can't discuss it openly; there's a stigma of shame in suicide and a tremendous sense of guilt. Somehow, someway, you let it happen. If only you had done or said things differently.

Suicide is more common than you think.

✗ Approximately 50,000 Americans kill themselves every year, leaving half a million survivors to mourn.

✗ Suicide is the third leading cause of death in the military.

✗ Five thousand teenagers commit suicide every year.

✗ Each year, between 100 and 300 physicians kill themselves—and female doctors have a three-to-four-times higher suicide rate than women in other professions.

A study of suicide at Rush Presbyterian-St. Luke's Medical Center, in Chicago, found four main character traits all suicide victims have:

1. Heightened anxiety, with frequent panic attacks and physical distress
2. Frequent alcohol and drug abuse
3. A hopeless view of the world, combined with a lack of interest in life and an inability to experience pleasure
4. A past history of suicidal tendencies

By its very definition, adolescence is a confusing time, especially in today's tumultuous aftershock world. Almost every teenager has, at least once, felt completely isolated and alone. At least once, he or she has experimented with alcohol or been severely depressed. In fact, a staggering 2 million American teenagers have already attempted suicide. If your teenager is

- Spending less and less time with friends,
- Overeating or not eating enough,
- Performing poorly in school,
- Moping around the house,
- Displaying poor grooming habits,
- Acting abusively and violently, or
- Crying frequently,

it's vital for you to seek professional help immediately. Suicide can be prevented.

What about people who witness a suicide? The aftershock repercussions can be enormous. In his work with suicide witnesses, David N. Hayes found a great deal of unresolved grief reactions, including an inability to form new, warm, and trusting relationships and a chronic, pervasive guilt. Suicide witnesses wear their aftershock guilt like a second skin; they refuse to give it up because it is all they have. They never got a chance to say good-bye.

Janice, a bright, attractive twenty-five-year-old secretary, is a case based upon a report from David Hayes. She had gone to her mother's home for a visit—and found her hanging from a rope in the basement. At first she denied the death; her family refused to acknowledge death by suicide. Janice took over many of her mother's roles; she became the caretaker for her two brothers and sister. It wasn't long before aftershock set in, with recurring nightmares, lack of concentration on the job, a loss of appetite, and insomnia. When she began to grow terrified that she too would commit suicide, Janice sought help. She joined a support group for suicide witnesses and eventually, through discussions, understanding, and therapy, began to see herself as a survivor, not a victim. Today, she no longer fears that she will kill herself.

But a person doesn't have to witness the suicide of a close family member to develop aftershock. Recently train engineers in New Jersey witnessed several teenage suicides. They saw the youngsters jump on to the tracks, and they were helpless to pull the brakes in time. These workers have begun to exhibit severe anxiety before, during, and after their eight-hour shifts.

Suicide has become an aftershock reality in the 1980s, a fact of contemporary life many of us will know intimately—whether it be as the victim, his or her close friend or relation, or a witness.

FATE AND TRAGEDY

I again saw under the sun that the race is not to the swift, and the battle is not to the warriors, and neither is bread to the wise, nor wealth to the discerning, nor favor to man of ability, for time and life overcame them all. (Ecclesiastes 9:11)

Thousands of years ago, people understood that life and fate were sometimes unfair, that we don't always get what we deserve, that we are not always happy. Life is a constantly changing road, but one we can follow with strength if we understand the impact of its signs, the pressure points that can stand in our way.

PRESSURE POINT TWENTY ONE: PERSONAL ILLNESS

We can eat right and exercise. We can get enough sleep and learn how to moderate our stress. But even with all our precautions, illness can strike. And it can be terminal.

Here is an actual monologue from a patient who discovered he had cancer.

I know that very early on and for a very brief period of time, I had the feeling that oh my God, I'm not going to be able to enjoy pizza, or beer, or baseball games, but then I realized so what. . . . The enjoyment of those forms of entertainment is a very conscious state. I am not going to be conscious, therefore I will not know that I am not experiencing that kind of thing. So death is very easy to deal with for me anyway. The problem I'm having is with dying . . .

How do we come to terms with death? We talk about it in a therapeutic environment; we have support groups; we try to accept our condition and our fear. (See the six stages of acceptance in Chapter Four.) But it is the survivors, the ones who will be around later, who "suffer," as in the above example, from being conscious. They are the targets for long-term aftershock. Here is the wife of the above patient talking with myself and Dr. Glicksman:

QUESTION: How did it hit you when finally the reality your husband has cancer that may, that will kill him? . . . Did you think 'My God I can't believe this? This is unreal, I wish I'd wake up'?
PATIENT'S WIFE: I'm getting closer in starting to believe. Oh, I could rationally talk about this and accept it and listen to the doctors and understand it, but I never really believed it. No and that's . . . I don't know if I'm even to the point yet that I really, really do in fact believe that he's going to die.

Unlike this woman, heart attack victims believe in their mortality too much. They cannot escape the feeling that they are going to die soon. Witness a different patient who had talked to both Dr. Glicksman and myself.

PATIENT: I woke up sometime around 3:00 and 3:30 in the morning. . . . I knew exactly what I was having and I got up and went into the living room with a pad of paper and pencil and figured out all the insurance that I had, all of the money that we had saved and the equity on the house and the whole thing, so that I knew exactly what we had financially and where my wife and children would stand. I was fairly confident that they would be able to get by with what was left and went back in and kissed my wife goodbye.

112

This man was one of the lucky ones. He did not die. He recovered and today leads a normal life. But not every recovered heart attack victim does as well. A case in point involves Edgar, a man who had a heart attack at thirty eight. It was a minor attack, but he spent the rest of his life terrified that it was going to happen to him again. He didn't take any risks in his job or his life and since the attack has actually spent over forty years on eggshells, wasting his life in fear—a terrible symptom of aftershock. But Edgar is not alone; a study conducted by Murray A. Brown, M.D., found that after a catastrophic illness like a heart attack, there is an inherent physical weakness and lack of control —at least during the time of recuperation. Unfortunately this very real weakness brings with it a decrease in self-esteem and confidence, and, in turn aftershock's anxiety and depression.

The best medicine for people who have recovered from their illness is to return to work, to get back into the mainstream. But many cannot. Their aftershock translates into a back-to-work phobia, which can be perpetuated by poor performance and long-term unemployment. Since many victims believe that work was the cause of the heart attack in the first place, returning to the job may only set off another attack, this time one that could be fatal.

Another test of courage is the trial of parents whose children have a life-threatening disease. Familiar in hospitals are women who come and stay with their critically ill children, refusing to give in to the illness, refusing to give up hope. Describing these "hospital mothers," Monica Dickens wrote in her book, *Miracles of Courage* (Dodd, Mead and Co., 1985) "Hope keeps parents going. When the doctor tells a mother, 'We have only a five percent chance of winning,' the number 95 does not appear in her mind. She is looking at the five, upward toward life." And indeed there are many cases where that hope has brought a child through the worst to live a healthy, long life.

An upcoming operation is another major potential cause of aftershock. After all, it goes against our primal instincts of survival to think of a surgeon's incision, even if it is for our health. A patient of mine named Jim had been apprehensive before his surgery for prostatic cancer. After several sessions, he finally accepted the necessity of the operation and it was a success. But six months later, he was breaking into tears unpredictably at his desk, at the dinner table, even during a comedy movie.

IF SOMEONE YOU LOVE IS SICK AND NEEDS YOUR CARE. . . .

1. Don't question your strength. Simply do what you have to do every day.

2. Try to find some free time. Whether it's an hour of exercise, watching TV, or listening to a record, it's important to nourish yourself in order to nourish others.

3. Try to feel hopeful. If you are religious, go to church. Read inspirational books. Meditate.

4. Keep your day-to-day routines up. Even the smallest errand is an accomplishment. It helps you stay in control of yourself.

5. Don't hesitate to ask for help—and don't hesitate to give it. Sharing brings strength. As a parent who suffered through her child's battle with a debilitating illness said: "The love that pours in is the saving grace of tragedy." (From *Miracles of Courage* by Monica Dickens, Dodd, Mead and Co., 1985.)

A fear of surgery can have disastrous results. A case in point is Margaret, a middle-aged woman who discovered a growth on her breast. She refused to see a doctor; she denied the node's existence. After all, she felt perfectly fine; she looked well. The truth was that Margaret's mother had died from cancer at an early age, and she was terrified that the same fate would befall her. But Margaret's denial, her unresolved grief over her mother, and her fear brought about the worst. For Margaret aftershock resulted in death. Eventually she began to feel ill and was forced to see a physician. The growth that could easily have been removed in the cancer's early stages had spread. It was too late.

A person learns to adjust to a chronic illness. If you get bronchitis every winter, you will make sure you wear a scarf. If you are prone to asthma, you will relocate to a drier climate. If you get frequent yeast infections, you will eat more yogurt. If your eyesight is fading, you will adjust to large-type books once the condition is accepted and understood.

But psychosomatic illnesses are not as clear cut. As a French doctor said, "The organs weep where the heart cannot." Ulcers, colitis, migraines, fatigue, these and many other illnesses may have their roots in stress. Psychosomatic problems do not have to be chronic; they can be cured by treating the emotional aftershock that caused them. Joan, for example, had been a two-pack a day smoker for years. When she finally took the positive step of quitting, she developed colitis. Her illness debilitated her, and consequently she went back to cigarettes, after which her colitis disappeared. If Joan had been treated for the stress that led to her smoking in the first place, she would never have developed colitis. And she would have remained a nonsmoker.

PRESSURE POINT TWENTY TWO: DEPRESSION

Clinical depression can be a disease unto itself, not just a result of aftershock. A life event can set it off. A person's family history can set it off. Stress can set it off. As Dr. William Z. Potter told *Business Week:* "Depression is like a fever. It's a nonspecific response of the brain to a variety of environmental and metabolic stresses."

Like TB a century ago, depression is the stress disorder of the 1980s. In actuality, clinical depression has been around for many years, but it was masked by other diseases, by pestilence, and by the effects of hard times. In today's world, depression is more prevalent than ever. Every ten years there is a marked increase in the number of cases—a direct correlation to the complexities of modern life.

The symptoms of depression include:

- Weight change
- Erratic sleep habits
- Lack of focus
- Self-deprecation
- Lack of energy
- Lack of interest in life
- A feeling of overwhelming sadness
- Suicidal thoughts

Depression is insidious. Minor symptoms can go away in six months, but the longer the depression, the worse it gets, and the greater the chances of it recurring. Once you are clinically diagnosed as depressive, you must face the fact that only medication and therapy will provide a cure. And if left untreated, depression can result in suicide.

Fact: Depression can make you accident prone. Witness the case of a depressed woman who had lost her husband. Three months after his death, although a careful driver all her life, she was involved in a near-fatal car crash on her way home from work.

Fact: Contrary to popular opinion, women do not suffer from depression more than men. But a study of forty-five depressed mothers of preschool children found that once women *are* depressed, their condition is more difficult to diagnose. They are better able to go about their everyday routines than men. They will not discuss their depression openly for fear of rejection. Their symptoms, in many cases, are less extreme and often reflect normal behavior. They receive less sympathy and support; their families tend to deny the depression.

Fact: Depressives are still not trusted at home or in the workplace. Witness the man who was not hired for an executive spot because he had been hospitalized for depression—or the husband who refused to believe his depressed wife was suffering from a real disease.

Theodore J. Arneson, the president of a Minnesota-based corporation, had five bouts of depression since the early sixties. Because of its stigma, Arneson never talked about his condition until 1981. Now, he'll discuss his depression with anyone and everyone fighting for the rights of depressive employees. He told *Business Week,* "Something has to be done. Depression is a major tragedy, people lose jobs and families."

Life is difficult enough without having to endure a handicap that can be cured. To operate at less than your full potential and faculties is a needless tragedy and an unnecessary pressure point. Today's depression not only can be treated—it must be. For the depressive the promise of the future is at stake.

PRESSURE POINT TWENTY THREE: ACCIDENTS

Depression and other aftershock conditions can cause accidents. A man who has just lost his spouse might drive his car into a tree.

A woman who just lost her job might break an ankle on the ski lift. A mother whose son is in the hospital might slip on the kitchen floor. And it's not only adults who suffer—studies show that children under personal and family stresses (such as tension with their parents, marital discord, or their parents' neglect) are more likely to have accidents.

But accidents *themselves* can cause aftershock as well. Consider two cases based upon cases presented in Dr. C. B. Scrignar's book on PTSD. Carl, for example, a successful businessman in his early fifties, was used to traveling a great deal. But en route to Los Angeles one morning, he was in a plane crash. Carl survived with only minor physical injuries, but three months later he developed aftershock, complete with nightmares, insomnia, lack of concentration, and sexual dysfunction. He and his wife grew apart. He grew anxious whenever he heard a plane overhead and he refused to fly again. His aftershock ultimately cost him his job.

Then there is the case of George, who fell off a ladder. He was stunned by his fall, but aside from a very minor backache and some bruises, he was fine. But six months later he too succumbed to aftershock. His symptoms manifested themselves in physical pain. He had constant aches and pains; he wore a back brace on and off. George spent his days going from doctor to doctor and always getting a clean bill of health. He refused to seek psychological help and his trauma is still very much alive today, thanks to a continuing lawsuit he has filed against the ladder company.

An accident victim is not the only one to fall prey to aftershock. A woman who saw a man run over by a car reacted by shaking. Several months later she found it impossible to cross the streets without help.

And from the pages of history, comes a case dated 1882. A man working in a telegraph office witnessed a train smash right through the wall. He was unharmed; he merely stood there in stunned amazement. But he, too, developed aftershock and later received payment for disability.

PRESSURE POINT TWENTY FOUR: SEXUAL EXPERIENCE

Regardless of how precocious or sophisticated today's teenagers might be, losing their virginity remains an important and sensitive issue. Witness the success of Norma Klein's books for young adults or movies like *St. Elmo's Fire*.

Once upon a time, men rarely married the woman with whom they had their first sexual experience, but women almost always married their first sexual partner. Because society dictated that women stay virginal (or at least look the part) until they were married, they were much more vulnerable during their first experience. More times than not, they would fall madly in love with their first partner. But these marriages were usually less than made in heaven—based, as they were, on inexperience and fleeting sexual attraction.

Even today, where sexual exploration is a given before making a larger commitment, women still fall in love with their first lovers. Alice met Sam in college, on the way to art history class. There was an immediate attraction, and after a few weeks they made love. For Sam it was great; for Alice it was love. She couldn't get enough of him, even though he had never made a commitment, verbally or otherwise. She became obsessed, and in her own version of the movie *Fatal Attraction*, began to follow him and his other dates. Ultimately Alice met another man and stopped obsessing about Sam. But she was never able to experience the same sexual feeling she had had.

Sex *is* different today. AIDS, sophistication, and cynicism have all taken their toll of romance, sometimes with disastrous results.

Homosexuals have always to fight the world, but today, because of AIDS, they are being preyed upon even more. In fact, 72.3 percent of a group of Minneapolis homosexuals suffered verbal harassment, 23.2 percent suffered from physical assault, 5.9 percent were raped because they were homosexual, and 66.6 percent kept silent about their abuse.

It's important to keep in mind that a person in a state of aftershock will always be in an identity crisis—regardless of the trauma that set it off. He or she will be defined not only by the crisis but by the response of others. Feeling lost, feeling adrift, feeling insecure, all are symptoms of crisis. And not knowing who you are goes right to the primal core, your sexuality.

PRESSURE POINT TWENTY FIVE: UPSWINGS OR WHEN GOOD THINGS HAPPEN TO GOOD PEOPLE

In the New York City area, there is a club that meets once a month in a suburban house. The members sit on folding chairs and eat bagels and tuna fish while, outside, the Mercedeses and Jaguars are lined up

Sex therapists are seeing a new problem among their patients: a lack of interest in sex. Called a "yuppie" disease because it's prevalent among young hard-working professionals, there are many theories for its origin—from a virus to poor time management, from lack of real communication to stress. Basically, when two people are so wrapped up in their working lives, it's difficult for them to wind down once at home. Excitement, pleasure, power plays, exercise—all find a place during the working day . . . which usually ends long after prime-time TV has begun.

The cure? Setting aside some time each week for each other, to talk about your personal goals and dreams—or simply to be together with no talk at all. If you or your partner find that you continue to remain "keyed up" and uninterested in sex, it would be wise to seek the help of a therapist.

waiting. It's an exclusive club; membership is by invitation only. This is the Millionaires Circle Club, a self-help group for lottery winners. As one member, a former accounts-payable coordinator, told *The New York Times:* "It's very relaxing to be with people in the same exact situation. I'm always conscious of talking to normal people and saying something that might sound horrible." The members call it "the post-lottery depression syndrome"—and they are not being self-indulgent. As I have discussed in Chapter Three, positive life-changing events have their own traumatic value, their own aftershock. For these winners, it is the outside world, ready to exploit them. They are alone, experiencing the "loneliness of the long-distance runner" like the boy in high school who was an award-winning student, but who had no dates, or the woman who had a nose job to look beautiful—and found her life as lonesome as before.

Whether it's inheriting a lot of money or moving to a better neighborhood, change brings its own stress timetable. It can take six months for people to adjust to a new home, especially if children are involved.

One has only to look at comedian Freddy Prinze, the Puerto-Rican star of the hit television series, *Chico and the Man.* He managed to leave his tough ghetto neighborhood and find fame and fortune in Hollywood, only to fatally shoot himself at the pinnacle of his career. Guilt, anxiety, fear—they also crop up in good things.

PRESSURE POINT TWENTY SIX: DOWNWARD MOBILITY OR WHEN BAD THINGS HAPPEN TO GOOD PEOPLE

An overheard conversation revolved around a group of young adults. They were joking about starting a self-help group for people who grew up with money but don't have it any longer. They would sit around and wax sentimental about the china they once had, the trips they took, the clothes they once wore.

The point is that tightening one's belt is no joke. According to statistics, baby boomers on the whole cannot afford the house they grew up in. Inflation, higher taxes, plus a college education that ill-prepared them for the real world has left many adults in their thirties and forties confused and prime candidates for aftershock.

Whether it's from a divorce, where statistics have shown that income is cut approximately in half for both parties; a loss of a job that results in less money and less self-esteem; or moving from a three-bedroom house to a cheaper apartment downward mobility can hurt. It can cause depression, anger, recurring nightmares, sadness—all the counterproductive symptoms of aftershock. Instead of helping you work on getting out of a mess, these symptoms keep you down and push you further down.

PRESSURE POINT TWENTY SEVEN: IS THAT ALL THERE IS?

> In this world there are only two tragedies—one is not getting what one wants, and the other is getting it. (Oscar Wilde)

It's the malaise of the eighties, a symptom of our times, a disease of the heart. It's the hollow end of materialism. It's called boredom—a trauma for today. Boredom is a symptom of stress and a stressor itself, and it affects more people than you might think. Take Jean. When she was a teenager she dreamed of marrying a doctor. She wanted a tall, handsome man that would take care of her; she wanted to be wife and mother and have money. Today, it looks as if her dreams have come true. She is an attractive, forty-five-year-old woman with a beautiful home on lots of land, two children who are growing up well, a loving husband, and complete financial security. She has everything she ever thought she wanted—and she is miserable.

Jean is a perfect example of an underachiever, someone who early in life decided what they wanted but aimed too low. The suburban married life was not what Jean really wanted, it was what society told her she wanted. It reflects society's values, not hers. Consequently, she is not satisfied, even though she seems to have everything she could want. Through therapy, she is learning what she is capable of and what she would like to do. She is currently going back to school, and her family is planning a move to the city.

On the other side of the coin is the overachiever, typically the yuppie, who also has everything he or she supposedly wants—but still wants more. A case in point is Elise. She is head of the marketing division of a high-tech Fortune 500 firm. She makes a six-figure salary that is not affected by the crash; she travels first class to luxurious hotels all over the country; she has an exquisite condo in a good section of Boston; she can buy the best.

But who has time for relationships? She is so busy working that she can't possibly handle personal commitment. As with so many other people in her position, there is no time for relationships. Things take on a value, the bigger and pricier the better. Love is replaced by objects that, because they can never be nourishing or fulfilling in and of themselves, are never enough.

Only when you achieve a balance between overachieving and underachieving will you be able to handle the slings and arrows of a most subtle form of aftershock.

THE FAMILY CIRCLE

When aftershock strikes, the whole family gets involved. Here are the unique pressure points of all-encompassing aftershock. It happens in the best of homes.

PRESSURE POINT TWENTY EIGHT: WORKAHOLIC FAMILIES

Home and career: The Great Unbalancers. On one hand, we want a family—children and a nourishing home life. On the other, we love our jobs and need our salaries to live.

The world where the husband went off to work while the wife stayed home to tend the hearth has gone the way of *Leave It To Beaver*. Today, an estimated 40 million of American homes are two-career households, with both parents working in responsible jobs and spending less time at home. The results are less parental supervision, less time together, and stress brought home from the office—all of which spells trauma. A magazine editor has a child who refuses to read. An investment banker has two teenagers involved in drugs. A pediatrician has children who refuse to talk to her—and the list can go on.

In a study of eighty-six upper-middle-class families, Professor Jeanne Brett and Sara Yogev found that women handled the dual problem of home and career better than men. The women were able to cut down their work time and make sacrifices for their families with a minimum of fuss. The men, however, made fewer changes in their schedules and felt more stress.

PRESSURE POINT TWENTY NINE: ALCOHOLIC FAMILIES

One out of every ten Americans suffer from alcoholism—leaving their scars on approximately 28 million children. Whether from fear of physical abuse or as a result of complete neglect, these children are forced at a very early age to take over major responsibilities at home. Deprived of dependable love and security, they grow up with

- Poor self-images
- A need for constant approval—that's always unfulfilled
- Tremendous guilt
- Repressed anger
- A sense of profound shame

It happens in the best of homes, and it's happening more and more in these stressful times. One child spends her evenings dragging her father home from the corner bar. Another stores food in her bedroom so she will have something to eat when her mother stays out drinking. And yet another child locks the door to her room on the nights her father drinks, so he won't beat her up.

Because they usually keep their family's affliction under wraps, children of alcoholics never get a chance to express their traumatic pain. Instead, they may go from one bad relationship to another in a downward spiral of self-destruction. And more times than not, they will become alcoholics themselves.

Today, alcoholism is recognized as a family disease, and there are

BALANCING A HOME AND A CAREER

Abraham Lincoln could have been talking about the eighties when he said, "You can't please all of the people all of the time—but you can please some of the people some of the time." When it comes to balancing a home and a career, you just can't do it all. Here are some tips to accomplishing some things, balancing some work and some play, and pleasing some people—especially yourself and your family—each day:

⚡ **Prioritize.** Computers now have software that does the work of an efficient manager, assistant, and filer. Check into them. They can keep your mind clear and your work organized.

⚡ **Be flexible.** If there's a week where you simply can't miss that meeting, make it up to your family a week later—and vice versa.

⚡ **Delegate.** Both at home and in the office, sharing responsibility means less time on drudgery and more time on challenge or entertainment.

⚡ **Open the door to both worlds.** Let your family see where you work. Discuss your work. By letting your family participate in your career, they won't be as resentful when you have to change plans. And their understanding will go a long way in aiding your performance during the day. Both your home and your office are crucial elements in your life. They shouldn't be separated as if they were alien worlds.

⚡ **Let go.** Whether you're in the midst of a sales pitch in the conference room or whether you're packing up for a family picnic—give it your full attention. Dwelling on your family when you're at work or dwelling on your work when you're at home is not only distracting—it's harmful to you and both your worlds.

almost 4,000 support groups offering alcoholics and their families un-understanding and help.

PRESSURE POINT THIRTY: PHYSICAL AND SEXUAL ABUSE IN FAMILIES

Fact: Approximately 1,300 children died of abuse or neglect in 1986 alone. Sexual abuse is a very real problem and an aberrant symptom of these aftershock times. The most notorious case in recent years in-volved a lawyer in New York's Greenwich Village. For years, the lawyer had allegedly terrorized his lover, his illegally adopted six-year-old daughter, and his illegally adopted infant son. It was not until the little girl died from his abuse that the story came to the country's attention. Then, and only then, the gruesome details came out, triggering after-shock in neighbors who hadn't realized the extent of the problem, teachers who felt they hadn't done enough, and government agencies that hadn't seen the signs.

More times than not, children who are abused become abusers when they grow up or take the law into their own hands. Witness the story of a sixteen-year-old girl from a typical suburban town. Her father had been sexually abusing her for years, as her mother watched help-lessly. No help was forthcoming; this was a private family affair. Fi-nally, unable to take it anymore, she hired a friend to kill her father. He did.

Privacy is the key factor here. People respect the privacy of oth-ers. Families tend to keep their shameful problems private. Less pri-vacy and more openness can stop this pressure point from reaching such tragic proportions.

PRESSURE POINT THIRTY ONE: AMBIVALENT HOMES

Every child needs to feel loved. But in ambivalent homes the signals get mixed. Children may feel love—but they also feel hate. Conse-quently these children grow up with a great deal of anxiety and uncer-tainty. They are never quite sure of their acceptance in the outside world, and they can never express even minor differences of opinion without suffering the pain of aftershock.

Ironically, ambivalent homes stop children from learning the les-sons of ambivalency: those shades of gray that are a part of life. Take Pam. Her mother hadn't expected to get pregnant when she did. On an unconscious level, she resented Pam for constricting her freedom and preventing her from living the life she wanted. But Pam's mother couldn't accept this hate; she felt horribly guilty and expressed it by acting in a completely opposite way. She showered Pam with love, almost suffocating her in her protectiveness. But Pam was a sensitive child. She detected the hate and unconsciously reciprocated it. She grew up with it all bottled up inside and passed along the same unexpressed feeling to *her* child.

In her book, *The Drama of the Gifted Child* (Basic Books, 1983) Dr. Alice Miller explains how this traumatic ambivalency prevents kids from having a normal childhood. These children are so eager to feel their parents' love that they never take the chance to rebel. Instead, they try to make their parents feel better; they unconsciously assume a nurturing role and keep their resentment under lock and key. It is only years later that it comes out, in such aftershock symptoms as depression, psychosomatic illness, and panic attacks.

This same ambivalence can be seen in depressed households or in homes where marriages are breaking up. It is a subtle but deadly pressure point that can seriously affect your future health and happiness.

Robert Louis Stevenson said, "To be what we are, and to become what we are capable of becoming is the only end in life." To overcome these personal pressure points is a step toward that goal, a victory of strength and resilience.

But there is another place where trauma can strike: on the job. Because stress is so prevalent in the business world today, these pressure points deserve their own chapter.

CRIMES IN THE FAST TRACK:

THE BUSINESS WORLD

*Life is not a matter of holding good cards
but playing a poor hand well.*
—ROBERT LOUIS STEVENSON

THE SIXTIES WERE THE WE DECADE; THE SEVENTIES were the Me Decade. The eighties? Think "Re" Regrouping, Rethinking, and Retrenching in the Corporate World. Nowhere are the vast changes in our daily lives seen as much as in business: 2.8 million employees in Fortune 500 companies have been let go in the past ten years. Countless others have gotten used to smaller paychecks, more responsibility, fewer hours in the day, and an environment of insecurity. The name of the game is downsizing, and it's becoming a new way of life, a new category of trauma that is hitting us more and more where we live.

THE BOTTOM LINE

In the film *The Secret of My Success*, Michael J. Fox comes to New York City to make it in the business world. He walks to a towering skyscraper to report to work, his expectations high. He enters the office of his new boss for the first time—and the last. His boss turns to him and says "Hostile takeover. Ninety percent of the people in this building are out on the street. You are one of those 90 percent. Tough break."

Comedy can reflect life. Perhaps it doesn't happen in such a dramatic way, but hostile bids and conglomerate mergers have made the business world as insecure a place as the eye of a tornado. Even in the above movie, the board's answer to fighting hostile bids was skimming costs. Budgets are being slashed across the country because all extra money is needed to prevent the dreaded takeover.

But changes are in the air. Within the next few years, there will be a switch. Competing companies have already cut costs as much as they can; prices are as low as they can go and still produce a profit. Quality will soon be the new magic element; it's the only way to combat the competition both abroad and at home.

And now that the dust is beginning to settle, companies are looking to the employees who have survived, hoping to soothe battered, embittered egos. Stress is already costing American companies a good $150 billion a year in medical payments, productivity, new reduction and management plans, and workmen's compensation settlements. Stress is Big Business and causing Big Problems. Analysis is crucial to mergers and takeovers, of the stock market reverses, and the changing business climate.

PRESSURE POINT THIRTY TWO: CRY MERGER!

The term "corporate power" used to conjure up a picture of a despot sitting at the end of a long conference table, cutting off heads as he cut off the tips of his cigars. Today it's very different; corporate power is healthy. In fact, anyone in the corporate world who doesn't crave power won't have much luck moving up the ladder.

Conversely, the lack of power can make you neurotic—and losing control over your job situation can mean anxiety, panic, and fear that permeates every aspect of your life—at the office *and* at home.

That's exactly the disquieting scenario currently being played during corporate mergers across the country. Witness the story of Robert Hearsch, a former supervisor at Hughes Aircraft. He enjoyed his job very much, but when General Motors took over Hughes, he got demoted. The result, as he recounted to *Newsweek*, was a mild nervous breakdown and a divorce.

Another story: Kelly's advertising agency had merged with another; there had been talk of massive firings, but since the decisions were being made behind closed boardroom doors, no one knew for sure. Kelly felt lucky when she survived the first go-around. She was able to keep her copywriting job, but instead of the "glamour" accounts, she got the direct-mail dregs. Her disgruntlement increased when her new boss came in from the new agency. He was tyrannical. He didn't fire her, because of his own anxious fears of reprisal, but he made her life miserable. Soon there were fresh rumors that another round of firings were in the offing. Kelly felt out of control and anxious. She hated her job, but she was terrified to be without one.

Family-oriented companies, with their secure jobs for life, have become a myth of the past. Loyalty has gone out the window along with those long-term jobs. Today's business climate makes security impossible, and the result is stress. So much stress, in fact, that companies will be spending approximately $15 million on wellness programs within the next decade—with everything from diet and exercise clinics to biofeedback and relaxation sessions. One company has even instituted a t'ai chi program to soothe its employees' nerves.

The crucial element is control. With so many global decisions made among the few, the bulk of managers and workers have no say and no control, but because of all the cutbacks and layoffs, they do have more responsibility. And responsibility without control translates into stress.

Proof that people need control comes from a study of baboons done at Stanford University. Researcher Robert Sapolosky discovered that in a stable hierarchy the animals near the top were able to handle stress better than their subordinates because they had power. But in unstable hierarchies, as in today's tumultuous business world, the higher-ups had an even harder time handling stress than those lower down.

Employees must renew their sense of control. Hewlett-Packard, a company long recognized as one of the best to work for, understood

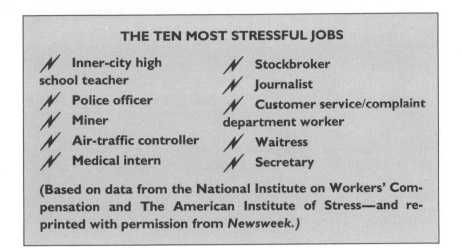

THE TEN MOST STRESSFUL JOBS

- Inner-city high school teacher
- Police officer
- Miner
- Air-traffic controller
- Medical intern
- Stockbroker
- Journalist
- Customer service/complaint department worker
- Waitress
- Secretary

(Based on data from the National Institute on Workers' Compensation and The American Institute of Stress—and reprinted with permission from *Newsweek*.)

this. The company had been going through a fierce competitive battle, especially with Far Eastern manufacturers. It had to buckle down; everyone took a pay cut, even the CEO. At the same time, Hewlett-Packard kept the research and development budget high. Even as it cut back, the company had the foresight to give growth and innovation a chance.

The most successful innovation came from Lee Iacocca. When he took over Chrysler, he didn't just cut salaries. He brought everyone together and made them feel like a part of the team. His "We're all in this together" theme did the trick. Everyone pitched in; everyone felt they had some control over their company's destiny.

PRESSURE POINT THIRTY THREE: BLACK MONDAY

It happened on a Friday in 1929—the stock market crash that was to be followed by the Great Depression. The government vowed it would never happen again. The power of the Federal Reserve was beefed up, insuring that banks would not run out of money. New regulations were set up on the stock market floor; trading had to be backed up with cash.

But times change. Rules are only obstacles to overcome. Traders began to buy and sell their stock options without money to back them up. Banks were forced to come up with the cash for huge recalls.

Trading itself was going wild, especially because of rampant and erratic insiders' tips. Salaries were soaring. Anyone on Wall Street was, according to Tom Wolfe *(The Bonfire of the Vanities,* New York: Farrar, Straus, and Giroux) a "master of the universe." Kids fresh out of school started with six-figure salaries. The sky was the limit. . . .

Until the storm came. On Monday, October 19, 1987, the stock market plummeted.

"Black Monday" has come and gone. The result? Massive retrenching, new laws and regulations, white-collar arrests for insider trading, and firing, firing, firing. Approximately 50,000 people will be out of work when the dust finally clears.

The most devastating fall was that of E.F. Hutton. The crash ruined the brokerage company, and it was merged with Shearson Lehman. The new regime immediately called for layoffs in what proved to be a massive bloodletting. Thousands were laid off under terrible circumstances. In one firing, the 300 members of E.F. Hutton's trading, investment banking, and stock research departments were shepherded into an auditorium and told en masse that they were fired. The man who had to make that announcement was later hospitalized for stress-related ailments. According to *USA Today,* he was told to have the employees clear their desks by 5:00 p.m. He refused and demanded one week.

Paranoia on the Street is rampant today. Theft, the handling of sensitive documents, ambiguous gossip, and insecurity: all make people lash out.

There is even a new successful firm to help new acquirers make a smoother transition, to help them handle their layoffs and firings more humanely. Not handled right, with outplacement counseling and good severance pay, the people fired might, as the president of the company told *USA Today,* "do everything they can ethically and unethically to screw 'em back."

CEOs, too, are feeling the pain of today's business traumas. E.F. Hutton's president had to pace the receptionist area of Shearson's offices while he waited to hear if the new kingpin was going to give him the axe. In total, all 18,000 E.F. Hutton employees were affected. Each one had to go for interviews at the new company to see if he or she still had a job.

Others on Wall Street have yet to lose their cool. There is still a lot of bravado around; people still feel they will be snatched up. The ones that have remained have rationalized the situation, deciding that the ones who got laid off just weren't the right stuff. But as one banker told *Glamour Magazine*, "Here are all these people who've gone through this process of convincing themselves they're worth all this money—thinking, 'I must be worth two, three, four hundred thousand dollars because somebody's willing to pay me that much.' But now the money isn't there anymore. . . . In the end, it really is a classical tragedy."

She might be right. With car payments, huge mortgages, and extravagant lifestyles to uphold, the pressure for many has yet to explode.

PRESSURE POINT THIRTY FOUR: TORNADO WATCH

A company man in a one-company town—it's the stuff of long ago. Today's business borders on the chaotic. The following section challenges your perception of the modern business climate where the rules have not only changed—they have intensified:

I. Geography Test

Myth: Mr. Grey was hired as a middle manager in a chemical engineering firm. He moved to the town near its corporate headquarters in Ohio. He bought a lovely home, sent for his wife and kids, and settled in for life.

Fact: Today, with mergers, acquisitions, and competition from abroad, companies can no longer offer the security they once did. People who have been employed for years are being laid off or offered early retirement. Companies are going under at a steady—and sobering—rate.

Myth: Chances are, if you get a job in a big city, you'll be staying for a nice long time. If a corporation has put down roots in New York, or Los Angeles, or Chicago, it won't be looking to relocate soon.

Fact: J.C. Penney, a long-time Manhattan resident, moved its corporate headquarters to Plano, Texas. The uproar caused so much stress that the company hired eleven new counselors. Previously, there had been only one. NBC, a New York City institution, was looking at property in New Jersey. And many of the sacrosanct Hollywood conglomerates have been checking out Disney's Orlando, Florida.

2. Global Implications have nothing to do with Middle America

Myth: Japan is essentially a tourist attraction. It would be fun to travel there on a vacation from my job.

Fact: The Far East has come into its own. In fact, the goals of imperialistic Japan as announced during World War II have become a reality: mass production, branches all over the world, and manufacturing plants even in America. Witness Honda or the combined forces of General Motors and Toyota.

Myth: Made in America is always best and always will be.

Fact: Made in Japan, once a label that was buried underneath products, has now come to symbolize quality. Many people consider Far Eastern goods and services, from cars to airlines, to be of higher quality than their American counterparts. We have become one big world, and we must continue to think better quality, better management, and fresh ideas in order to compete.

Myth: Even if one man takes over another's company, it's all in the family—or at least the American family.

Fact: Saatchi & Saatchi, a British-based organization has already taken over several American advertising agencies. Australian Rupert Murdoch is one of the giants of American communications.

3. All Dressed Up and No Place to Go

Myth: If I study hard in college and really apply myself, I'll take the business world by storm. Nothing can stop me if I work hard and learn fast.

Fact: Thousands of Wall Street brokers have already lost their jobs; most of them are under thirty, top students in their classes, and already living in overextended style. Thanks to all the mergers, takeovers, and budget cuts, there are fewer jobs out there for qualified people. To stop aftershock's most debilitating effects, AT&T started to spend a great deal of money two years *before* their divestiture to help their employees through the inevitable trauma. But even with their prevention strategy, morale today is still bad, and many employees have developed the "witness syndrome" reaction to trauma. When other people in other departments get the axe, they react as if they, too, are being asked to leave.

Myth: Work is a source of great pleasure. I can expect to enjoy job security, my colleagues, and the excitement of going to the office every day.

Fact: One corporate consultant told *Business Week* that "at least 45% of American managers suffer too much stress." The result? "They are becoming abusive, intolerant, and dictatorial."

Myth: Sure I have stress on my job. It comes with the territory. All I have to do is focus on the job, and maybe do a little jogging and eat more nutritionally to keep me on an even keel.

Fact: Fifteen percent of all corporate executives are suffering from so much stress they are becoming clinically depressed. Their families can't help. Parents and spouses tend to be emotionally supportive, trying to reassure with words: "Don't worry. You're terrific." They mean well, but their kind words fall on deaf ears. An executive's stress is primarily situation oriented. It has less to do with an inherent neurosis than it does with the extra workload at work, an unrelenting schedule, erratic job security, and a boss that is under just as much stress—and letting his or her anger and frustration filter down.

Add all these problems up and you have real cause for stress, real pressure points that can blow up into aftershock

PERSONAL PROFITS AND LOSSES

We've all seen how the larger corporate picture affects each one of us. But what about the more intimate changes, those events that hit us on a more one-on-one basis? What about promotions, demotions, early retirement, or a new career? Let's take a look now at our personal profits and losses. . . .

PRESSURE POINT THIRTY FIVE: PROMOTIONS

Ruth and Allen are a happily married couple who between them make over $200,000 a year. They enjoy a luxurious lifestyle, and though Ruth is a lawyer and Allen a graphic artist, they each understand the pressure and stress the other is feeling. Recently they both received partnerships in their respective firms. But all that prestige has translated into more time away from each other. Entering their new co-op one night, Ruth turned to Allen and said, "Gee, what a great apartment. I wonder who lives here?"

The fact is that doing well in the corporate world takes its own

> The seven characteristics of today's stress-filled corporate world:
>
> ⚡ Day-to-day insecurity over the possibility of losing your job
>
> ⚡ Too much work with fewer people to do it
>
> ⚡ No control over your own work destiny—even though you have tons of responsibility
>
> ⚡ Supervisors who are just as overworked and anxious as you—and who can't offer any support or help
>
> ⚡ Fewer options beyond the company's walls, fewer career opportunities, and fewer positions opening up elsewhere
>
> ⚡ Conflict between values of home, family life, and work and wanting to get ahead in an ethical manner and seeing others get faster and better results with amoral behavior
>
> ⚡ Uncertainty in a world where terrorism abroad can directly affect your company's profit and where overseas decisions can directly affect your work life in the States

aftershock toll. The anxiety can still build up. There is less time to enjoy the lifestyle you can now afford. And in many cases there is no time to enjoy a family, let alone start one. These trade-offs can hurt, even with the addition of prestige, power, and money.

Another potential aftershock zone comes from being promoted to a position where your predecessor had been fired. Randy's boss was fired and Randy was terribly upset. She liked him a lot. She was offered his spot and she took it because she could do the job well, she wanted to get ahead, and she had nothing to do with the firing. She even had her old boss's blessings. But two weeks after she started her new job, she began to wake up in the middle of the night with nightmares, crying "Oh no, not me too!" She not only felt guilty, she was also terrified that she would also be fired. Like the new bride whose husband cheated on his first wife, she faces the strong likelihood of it happening again.

Another promotion danger comes from a driving need to succeed, inherent in the overachievers I talked about in Chapter Eight. In those case histories, achievement didn't spell contentment; success only added to a sense of overwhelming responsibility. Overachievers often can't relate to people on a personal level; they can only think about getting ahead. A case in point is Joe, a man who is next in line for the presidency of his corporation. He wanted to spend more time with his family, and one Sunday, determined to spend the day with his wife and kids, he put the answering machine on and closed his study door. But he couldn't stop making lists and delegating jobs to everyone in the family, from preparing the lunches for a picnic to pinpointing the hours they would spend swimming, hiking, and eating. What should have been fun was spoiled when activities were resolved into a series of goals that had to be accomplished. Joe achieved his Sunday in the country with his family, but it felt like a full day's work.

The very personality traits that make a good doctor make for depression and stress: compulsiveness, conscientiousness, emotional control, and an ability to delay gratification. But more and more doctors are succumbing to their stress, and many of them have committed suicide. Why?

⚡ **Because every day they deal in life and death situations**

⚡ **Because their work schedules are unrelenting**

⚡ **Because there is so much responsibility on their shoulders**

⚡ **Because they have easy access to drugs—and the possibility of forming a habit while coping with the long hours, financial stress, and performance anxiety as interns and residents.**

Since a promotion is as much a traumatic event as any other crisis, chances are you will also experience an identity crisis. (See Chapter Eight.) How do you handle yourself on the new job? How will your former business colleagues handle your success? The unfamiliar is fraught with fear.

PRESSURE POINT THIRTY SIX: GETTING THE AXE

Item: In Riverside, California, a former Pacific Bell employee took several coworkers hostage and ruined the company's telephone equipment to the tune of $10 million.

Item: One man, who worked for a corporation in Des Moines, Iowa for twenty-one years, was laid off during an employee reduction. Ten months later, in February, 1988 he celebrated his fifty-sixth birthday by shooting himself.

Item: Not long ago, General Motors "offered" several of its managers early retirement. Four of them committed suicide.

Item: A Chicago-based editor for the Encyclopedia Britannica was so incensed about being fired that he sabotaged the publisher's computers, changing the names of historical people to Britannica employees and substituting Allah wherever Jesus appeared in the text.

Item: On April 7, 1988, the head of Merrill Lynch of Boston was shot and killed by a broker he had fired twenty-four hours earlier.

The bad news is that getting fired can hurt. The good news is that it no longer has the stigma it once had. Since 1980, 2 million people have been fired—and virtually none of them were fired for poor performance. No longer do people have to fidget when a prospective employer asks about the blanks on a resume or where the applicant is working today.

In fact, it is the ones who wield the axe who often pay. Not only do they have the guilt of initiating the divorce, but more and more, the people they are firing are getting even. The American Arbitration Association had more than 300 claims in 1986 alone, with over $29 million worth of damages for breach of contract. Lawsuits logged by the labor employment section of the American Bar Association rose a whopping 85 percent, and this figure doesn't even touch age-discrimination suits. In 1987 the amount of stress-related workmen's compensation claims reached an all-time high.

Today, employers go to seminars and receive counseling on how to fire. No longer can they simply leap up from behind their desk, as in 1940s movies, and roar "You're fired!"

Most of the people who do file a suit after getting fired earn over $40,000; they are the only employees who can afford the action, and they don't mind taking on the powers that be.

But even with the more open attitude, getting fired can hurt. And there are still people who face the trauma badly. As in the examples at the beginning of this section, getting fired can be enough to bring these people over the edge or to trigger aftershock symptoms from a previous event. Even deciding to file a lawsuit is a sign of aftershock. No matter how much you might win, you will always be branded as a troublemaker —and don't think you won't. Computer printouts of people who have filed malpractice suits are available to hospitals.

And if you are out of work for several months or longer, the stigma does return. A prospective employer starts to question your position. Why has it taken so long to find the right job? Why aren't you working yet? The fact is that there are still too many people out there and not enough jobs, and it is only going to get worse. As Robert J. Bies, an assistant professor of organization behavior at Northwestern University's Graduate School of Management, told the *New York Times*, "The mass layoffs of today will have a ripple effect on the whole hiring and firing process. . . . Executives will soon insist on a prenuptial agreement, one that spells out what the corporate divorce will be like."

Even people who eventually get hired can no longer feel secure. If it happened once, it can happen again. Loyalty to oneself comes first in today's environment of potential aftershock.

Being fired is a form of rejection. A piece of you has died, and you must go through a mourning state to come out unscathed. But believe it or not, many people do better *after* getting fired. If you had been in a job you hated, you could end up in one you like. The time off gives you a chance to explore other avenues and other careers. You can get to know your family better. It can be a real beginning. As other people who have been faced with trauma know, the best way to get through it is to stop feeling like a victim. You are a survivor—and a strong one too.

Even quitting can be fraught with anxiety. Along with your free choice comes the risk of the unknown. But when life gets too tough in the fast lane, the best way out is through the door. A case in point is Susan, a buyer for a large department store. The pressure was starting to get to her; she had one deadline after another and no time for herself. She was earning money she didn't have time to spend. For Susan, there was only one solution, to quit. She left the world of New York fashion

> **How do you know if your job is getting you stressed out?**
> 1. A faster heartbeat
> 2. Lower backache
> 3. Cravings for sweets in the middle of the day
> 4. Outbursts at your boss and colleagues
> 5. Lack of sleep the night before
> 6. Frequent upset stomach
> 7. Chronic absenteeism
> 8. A pervasive tired feeling
> 9. An inability to focus on the work at hand
> 10. Increased drinking or drug use
> 11. Biting your nails or rubbing your eyes too much
> 12. Obsessing about your job when you are not at the job
> 13. Having work-related dreams
> 14. Experiencing weight gain or loss
> 15. Constant complaints about the amount of work you have and the fact that nobody cares

and settled down in a small-town boutique where she could not only do the work she loved, but love the work she did.

PRESSURE POINT THIRTY EIGHT: RETIREMENT

In today's world, more and more people are being asked to take early retirement, which in many cases is a polite, and financially acceptable way of getting the axe.

Retirement, even for those who have planned and chosen it, can cause tremendous aftershock. After the gold watch and the banquet dinner, you are left with an empty space. Suddenly you no longer have to set the alarm. Suddenly the day-to-day concerns of the office don't concern you. Suddenly the people you spoke to every single day are no longer there. Suddenly you are driven to fill in the hours, before your thoughts turn to old age. Your routine, your values, your whole life have changed. It's no wonder retirement is considered one of the most stressful life-changing events.

PRESSURE POINT THIRTY NINE: CAREER SWITCH

Think of it: one day you are sitting at your desk, looking at your planner and trying to fit in everything you have to do that day. You turn and

> People who have become successful *after* retirement:
>
> ⁄⁄ Helen Hoover Santmyer became a bestselling author at eighty-eight with the publication of her novel " . . . *And the Ladies of the Club."*
>
> ⁄⁄ We can all hooray puree thanks to Carl G. Sontaheimer who invented the Cuisinart after retiring at fifty five.
>
> ⁄⁄ Marion Cunningham was a housewife until at fifty-seven she became a cookbook author, revising the famous *Fannie Farmer Cookbook.*
>
> ⁄⁄ When Maggie Kuhn retired at sixty-five, she became an activist, founding the powerful senior citizens' group, The Gray Panthers.
>
> ⁄⁄ Although his name might not be a household name, the product he invented in his sixties—after he retired—certainly is: Velcro fasteners. Today, in his eighties, George Demestral is healthy, wealthy, and wise.

look out the window—and realize you not only hate your job, you hate your career. And you've been feeling this way a long time . . .

It happens more than you think. Many people who own small businesses have turned out to be ex-ad men or ex-bankers or ex-buyers. An architect decides she wants to be a carpenter. A book editor turns into a writer. A writer turns into a marketing executive. A financier decides to open a bakery.

Knowing you are in the wrong career is as bad as the plight of the woman who wakes up one morning and realizes she is in the wrong marriage. It causes a great deal of stress—and aftershock symptoms ranging from irritability and anxiety to sleepless nights.

Changing careers means. . . .

A loss in pay—at least in the beginning

A possible move to another state or town

The loss of a whole circle of friends and colleagues

Taking a big risk: what if you're not successful?

Planning the move carefully, taking into consideration the ways your skills are transferable.

PRESSURE POINT FORTY: LOOKING FOR A JOB

You start out optimistic. You are going to hit the phones, pound the pavements, and get the job of your dreams. But it doesn't always work that way. First of all, if you are looking for a job, chances are you are already fraught with anxiety. Either you have been fired and your self-esteem is low, or you have decided to look for a new job and are (1) feeling guilty about calling in sick and (2) paranoid that someone from the office will find out.

More likely, things will go this way:

Rob got the call his last day at work. The headhunter said this was it; they liked his resume and they wanted to meet with him. Rob was excited. He had an early dinner with some friends, then went to sleep. Or rather, his head hit the pillow. Rob couldn't sleep. He was nervous. He couldn't stop thinking about the interview. The next day he drank some coffee to wake up and proceeded to feel even more anxious. By the time he reached his destination, his stomach was growling and his hands were sweaty. All his positive energy had turned into dust, his thoughts running the gamut from self-aggrandizement to self-destruction: "Will they like me? How can they like me? Of course, they'll like me. How could they not? Maybe they'll hate me."

But it doesn't have to be this way. Take a tip from some of the newly-fired Young Turks on Wall Street. They have confidence that someone else will want them. As one E. F. Hutton casualty told *Glamour Magazine*, "Finding a position that you want is not a process that occurs overnight. It takes at least a month if you're lucky, and sometimes two or three." Another example of confidence comes from a onetime public affairs director of a prestigious electronic firm. She lost her job and she was up front about her situation. "No one questioned the fact that I am without a job," she told the *New York Times*, and she fully expects not to be jobless for long.

If you are looking for a job right now, you can ease the aftershock symptoms by

[1] **Making a list of all the people you know. Seeing them all in print makes you realize you are not alone.**

2   Calling the people on your list. Let them know you are looking. Even if they are not in your field, it's possible that they know someone. And they will help give you important support and encouragement.

3   Following every lead; you never know.

4   Buying an oversized calendar and writing down all the calls you make on a given day, then putting those same names down for callbacks two weeks later. This way you have a plan of action that's immediately visible.

5   Easing your anxiety and guilt by doing at least one business-related task each day. Maybe it will just be one phone call. Maybe it will just be bringing your interview suit to the dry cleaners. It doesn't matter. Even the smallest action can stop your despair; you are doing something.

6   Using your free time exactly as you please. Whether it's seeing a friend for a drink, reading that book you always said you were going to get to, exercising, or just sleeping the afternoon away, nurturing yourself will help keep your spirits up.

7   Making a budget. It will help you feel in control of the situation. Figure out how much time you have to look before your funds run out. Think of some alternative plans so that even if the bottom does fall out, you have options. Remember, you are in control.

8   Not grabbing at the first you find. It's just as important to enjoy your job as it is to earn a living.

9   Keeping things in perspective. Looking for a job is not pursuing an impossible dream. It's not like wanting to live in a French chateau or planning a year-long cruise on your private yacht. The high employment figures are in your favor.

PRESSURE POINT FORTY ONE: WORK CONDITIONS

From your boss to the people you see every day, from the way the sun hits your office to the color of the office walls, your work environment is just as important as your job and your paycheck, when it comes to aftershock. And whether your work atmosphere is pleasant or traumatic begins with the boss—the parental figure, the controller, the one person who can be your fiercest ally or your worst nightmare come true.

    Doris worked for Rhonda, a boss who at first seemed very supportive. She always thought of Doris when she had an hour free; they spent several dinners discussing their personal lives. Rhonda always complimented Doris on her work, showing her appreciation with flowers or a typed-up memo. She kept telling Doris that she would go far. But then Rhonda started calling Doris up in the evenings, asking about mail and phone messages that had come in during the day. Soon she was calling Doris on weekends too. The job became a chore for Doris; Rhonda had become extremely demanding. When Doris tried to explain that she felt overworked, that she needed some time away from the office, she assumed that they would talk about it as they had in the old days. Instead, Rhonda started yelling; she began criticizing Doris for her lack of organization. Doris stuck it out for two more years, never getting the raise or the promotion she deserved. And when Doris finally got up her courage to quit, Rhonda refused to give her a good reference.

Why did Doris stay with someone who was obviously a terrible boss? Like many other people in the same situation, Rhonda managed to push all the right buttons, manipulating Doris with friendship before jumping in for the kill.

Relationships are complicated, especially bad ones. Often a terrible boss/victimized employee combination is merely a piece of a pattern that has been repeated since childhood. Perhaps Doris had never resolved her feelings about her mother; perhaps Rhonda saw Doris as the sister she had never gotten along with. Whatever the underlying problem, a relationship with a bad boss almost always results in anxiety and provides fertile ground for aftershock to grow.

In her book about competition among women in the office, entitled *Woman to Woman: From Sabotage to Support* (New Horizon Press, 1987), Judith Briles explains that many women blur the lines of business and friendship. But your boss is your boss is your boss, even if you do have a personal relationship. You can't work out your differences the way you would with a close friend. And the personal things you talk about can be used against you later on.

In her study of corporate executives, Dr. Suzanne Kobasa discovered that employees who liked their bosses and enjoyed working for them were less stressed. They felt better about themselves and their jobs.

Then there's the office itself. A badly constructed work area can cause tension. What if you have no privacy or if your desk is too

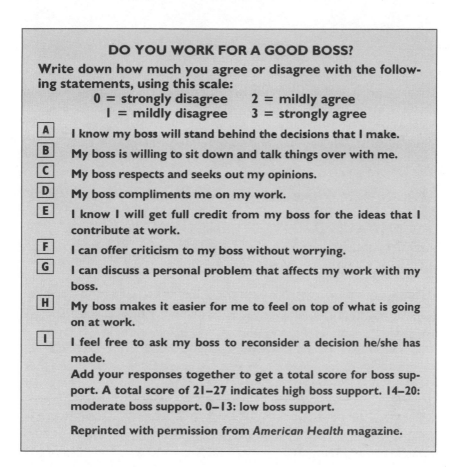

DO YOU WORK FOR A GOOD BOSS?

Write down how much you agree or disagree with the following statements, using this scale:

      0 = strongly disagree   2 = mildly agree
      I = mildly disagree   3 = strongly agree

A   I know my boss will stand behind the decisions that I make.

B   My boss is willing to sit down and talk things over with me.

C   My boss respects and seeks out my opinions.

D   My boss compliments me on my work.

E   I know I will get full credit from my boss for the ideas that I contribute at work.

F   I can offer criticism to my boss without worrying.

G   I can discuss a personal problem that affects my work with my boss.

H   My boss makes it easier for me to feel on top of what is going on at work.

I   I feel free to ask my boss to reconsider a decision he/she has made.

Add your responses together to get a total score for boss support. A total score of 21–27 indicates high boss support. 14–20: moderate boss support. 0–13: low boss support.

Reprinted with permission from *American Health* magazine.

crowded? The lighting can be too harsh or too soft. And more than anything else, the culture of your corporation can add to your trauma.

The Corporate Giants

These are the kings of the corporate empire, the Fortune 500s like AT&T and IBM, the companies with strict guidelines and family-oriented policies. Here you will find annual picnics and health clubs, top-of-the-line office equipment, and a focus on the bottom line. You will have cafeterias, counselors, stress-management workshops, excellent benefits, and more. These companies want your loyalty, and they want you to be happy. But don't come to work in unsuitable dress. Decorum is expected. Agree to follow the rules and you can be happy.

The Different Drummers

In these companies, individuality is encouraged. You can dress however you like as long as the work gets done. Everyone is approachable, from the president to the messenger. Corporate bureaucracies and regulations are anathema in these offices, but you will usually sacrifice salary for the more creative environment. Television, movies, publishing, and advertising are the fields where these companies flourish.

The Team Players

These are the companies that roar with spirit. They are the families of McDonald's, Mary Kay, and Chrysler. Here it's "all for one and one for all." If you work late one night, chances are the boss is working late right next door.

The Entrepreneurs

Go for it! is the slogan for these companies. They hear your ideas and they let you fly. Innovation is rewarded and you always share in the pie. An example here is 3M, a company that has long rewarded creativity with a step up the ladder—regardless of whether creativity is accompanied by management skills. If you come up with several great ideas, your chances of reaching the top are high. Think of Post-its. Those self-adhesive pads are a direct result of this kind of operating procedure.

These four corporate cultures are of course generalizations. Most companies are a combination of all four personalities, with one more prominent than the others. Think about the place where you work. If your personality fits into its culture, you are likely to work out any problems with a minimum of stress. If your personality is vastly different, it's time to make a change, before you have to pay the price in aftershock. Here are five strategies.

⚡ Analyze your anxiety. Is it coming from your office's layout? Does it have to do with your boss? Is it the culture? How would changing it affect your career?

⚡ If your problem is too much travel, make new arrangements. Perhaps you can fly one way to be on time for the meeting, but unencumbered you can take a leisurely train ride back. Maybe you can combine your business trip with a long weekend and enjoy a short vacation.

"BIG BROTHER" IS WATCHING

From clerks carrying clear plastic pocketbooks to roaming security guards, companies have long kept tabs on their own.

But thanks to advanced technology, office monitoring has entered the twenty-first century—with TV cameras, itemized long-distance telephone bills, reproduction machine loggings, and, more than anything else, computer productivity counting. In 1987, six million computer operators in America were monitored while they worked. "User friendly" gets a whole new meaning when companies record how many times an operator hits the keyboard and how long a computer is "down" and not being used by its operator.

✗ The value of money doesn't last long, especially in the business world. If you are working solely for the money, there will soon come a time when you are dissatisfied. A paycheck, like the value put on things, is ultimately hollow. If you can't find any other reason for working in your company, then it might be time to leave, before the paycheck hooks you into being "trapped."

✗ If your commute is getting you down, check out a move. Maybe you can live closer to your office.

✗ Make sure your anxiety is work related and that your office is not the trigger for a different trauma that happened in your life. And if you are feeling seriously anxious or depressed, get help!

A study of 200 highly stressed AT&T executives done by the aforementioned Dr. Kobasa found that half remained healthy during the months of divestiture and the other half succumbed to aftershock. Why? It had nothing to do with youth or money. It had nothing to do with position in the pecking order or with education. But it had everything to do with hardiness. The AT&T executives who stayed healthy were more committed to their work and themselves. They liked challenge and they felt in control of their own situation.

Two Harvard professors, Yerkes and Dodson, discovered that stress actually helps productivity—but only so far. After a certain point, stress will sabotage job performance dramatically. In a world where three quarters of us find our jobs stressful, it's important for us

GET A STRESS-FREE OFFICE WITH:

⚡ **A clear desk.** Think of your desk as a tool of your trade —a piece of machinery that enables you to process information. Keep only one project at a time on your desk; with less clutter, you'll be more focused and calmer.

⚡ **A "tickler" file.** Let your files remind you of the day's important meetings and your future commitments. Set up an accordian file organized by day and month. Simply throw in any memos, phone numbers, and lists that must be taken care of on a particular day. You can then forget about it until that date.

⚡ **A list of things to do.** Lists are great stress-reducers— even if they have to be revised. Seeing your commitments in black and white goes far in calming your scattered thoughts. Make your list the night before and, the next day, do your "worst" chore first. You'll feel great that you finished it and accomplished something—and you'll find the energy to keep going.

⚡ **Communication.** There's nothing worse than a closed door to keep imaginations going strong. Clear feedback, open channels of communication, and delegation of responsibility all go far in calming nerves . . . and keeping stress to a minimum.

⚡ **An attractive space.** A favorite picture, a flowering plant, soothing color on the wall, and a bouquet of sweet-smelling flowers can all go far to visibly reduce the stress of busy office life.

to build up our hardiness, or we will fall victim to poor performance and the pain of aftershock.

Current Events, personal shocks, business traumas—the life and times of our eighties world. Bernard Baruch once said, "Lost opportunity is man's greatest hell." In the next two sections, you will have the opportunity to seek help for your aftershock symptoms and prevent them from ever harming you and your loved ones again. Opportunity is knocking. Read on.

Too much stress? Here's some ways companies are trying to help you cope:

𝄢 Stress-reduction tapes. Some of these help you visualize peaceful, relaxing scenes—a trip on a sailboat, a deserted beach, a cool forest. Others will combine these visualizations with deep-breathing exercises and calming suggestions.

𝄢 Biodots. Remember the mood rings of the sixties and seventies? These adhesive tapes are the eighties office's answer. Temperature sensitive, these tapes show when blood isn't flowing properly to your hands and feet—which signals stress.

𝄢 Exercise classes. From yoga and t'ai chi to aerobics and Nautilus equipment, companies are becoming more and more savvy to the role exercise plays in reducing stress. By organizing exercise classes at the office, there's less excuse not to join in.

𝄢 Laugh Tracks. Capitalizing on the truism "laughter is the best medicine," a computer company has recently put out a program that flashes jokes on computer monitors for stressed-out workers.

𝄢 Wellness programs. These stress-management strategies hope to stop stress—and its rising cost—in its tracks with diet programs, quit smoking clinics, group therapy, self-hypnosis seminars, and workshops on different techniques for relaxing.

PART THREE:

AFTERSHOCK THERAPY

A BETTER LIFE IS WAITING

"I don't know why I waited so long to travel."

"I used to blame everybody else for things that were really all my fault."

"I stopped making excuses."

"For the first time, I really believed that life will not last forever. I have to do things now and stop waiting for another day."

"Time? It's a luxury none of us can afford."

LISTEN TO THESE PEOPLE. ONE OF THEM SUFFERED from breast cancer. One survived a plane crash. A third one came from an alcoholic home. Another survived the terrible loss of a loved one. Still another had become the head of a corporation and was forced to confront an atmosphere of nonstop pressure. Each and every one of them has experienced a life-changing event. Each and every one of them succumbed to aftershock months after their initial trauma. And each and every one of them sought help—and came out far better than before.

Yes, today's world is filled with trauma. As we have seen in Section Two, some of them are as timeless as life itself; whereas some are specifically an eighties phenomenon. But think of it: Without these stressful traumas, there would be no opportunity, no chance, as the above people can testify, to make our lives better. The stress of a life-changing event forces us to change. With the proper therapy, that change can be positive, offering us a wiser view of the world, a new understanding of the people around us, a rare glimpse of ourselves and our destructive behavior in a clear, focused light. Therapy can help us move forward—toward a more capable and resilient future.

A crisis is a true window of opportunity. In the words of Bertrand Russell: "It's not the experience that happens to you, it's what you do with that experience."

There is life—a better life—after aftershock.

THE DYNAMICS OF CRISIS

A crisis changes things dramatically. Defenses are down; you are more open and vulnerable. In fact, the very crisis that is hurting you provides the fuel for the return to health. You are driven to change to eliminate the pain. Growth is much faster than in more orthodox therapeutic situations.

Several decades ago, psychologist Abraham Maslow developed a hierarchy of needs that motivate us. At the bottom are our primal, basic wants: the food, warmth, and shelter we need to survive. Once we have satisfied these needs, we can move up to less physical needs. Here are our urges for love, self-respect, and good work. Above these needs is the rarefied level of self-actualization—where we are truly living up to our potential, our ego needs no longer driving us around in circles.

Unfortunately, today's world, with its bombardment of promises and setbacks, its day-to-day traumas, puts most of us in the middle level—searching for love, more satisfying work, less stress-filled environments. But self-actualization is not an impossibility. By clarifying your values, your beliefs, and your desires in an intense, focused setting, crisis-intervention therapy inspires growth.

As Antoine de St. Exupéry said in *Wind, Sand and Stars*: "The image lies asleep in a block of marble until it is carefully disengaged by the sculptor. The sculptor must, himself, feel that he not so much inventing or shaping the curve of a breast or a shoulder, as delivering the image from its prison." This is the role of crisis-intervention therapy —to set you free.

PSYCHOTRAUMATOLOGY

The reasons for existing are unique to each person. In order to survive the fury of a trauma, a purpose for living must be found and that purpose is defined by you. With the proper therapy, you can discover the why and how of your life.

The first and foremost task of a crisis-intervention therapist is to ease your present anxiety by desensitizing your memories of your trauma. Just as a young anorexic girl, weak from lack of food, must first be given nutritional supplements before therapy can work, so must an aftershock victim get relief from his or her anxious, depressed symptoms before growth and understanding can take place.

Once your anxiety is eased, you can begin to understand and accept what has happened. Armed with that knowledge, your symptoms will start to fade, and the catapulting event will begin to find its way back to its rightful time and place. The event will become integrated with your "cognitive map," (that is, the way you look at the world, and you will ultimately gain a *new,* point of view, wiser and stronger.

This is where psychotraumatology, a new branch of biopsychiatry, comes in. Combining medicines that treat—not mask—your problems with both conventional individual and group therapies and newer, less orthodox methods, it ensures proper diagnosis and rapid crisis-intervention treatment. You not only reduce the impact of the trauma, you gain insight and psychological growth. From that "block of marble" emerges a new you, whole and complete, a person who has mastered the slings and arrows of outrageous aftershock.

FROM THE ABYSS TO THE LIGHT

As the medical director of Fair Oaks Hospital in Summit, New Jersey, I have seen the principles of psychotraumatology work time and again —from the mildest cases to the most severe. Throughout my career, I have had the privilege of analyzing and studying crisis intervention and of putting my ideas into practice. Through my long years of trial and error, I have developed twenty principles of crisis intervention that must be present for maximum results. I hope they will help you understand the dynamics of aftershock therapy, as well as aid your search for a therapy that works. Let's begin.

Principle one: Healthy, positive personality traits are emphasized. As we have learned, a life-changing crisis will always precipitate an identity crisis. Not only do you experience the pain of your trauma, you can also expect a loss of self-esteem, a feeling that you are a terrible person, a victim in a heartless world. But all is not bleak. If you have had solid friendships in your life, you will make new friends—despite moving to a strange new town or losing someone close to you. If you have been able to do the good work that has led up to your promotion, chances are you will continue to do that good work in your new role. The statistics are in your favor—despite the negative feelings you are experiencing. Good crisis-intervention therapy will help you logically and emotionally see this healthier side.

Principle two: Crisis therapy does not last forever. One of the ways crisis intervention differs from other, more traditional forms of therapy is its restricted time frame. You and your therapist are working quickly toward a common goal: relief from aftershock and an ability to live in a trauma-ridden world. This limited therapy forces you to rely more on your family and friends and less on your therapist—which in turn aids your adaptability to the world at large.

Principle three: A social support system is encouraged. In order to rely more on your friends and family, you need to develop close, *supportive* ties outside the therapist's office. Why are supportive ties stressed? Think about it: If you surround yourself with people who always seem to avoid you, you will become paranoid. If you are always put down by your family and friends, you will have little self-worth. But if you surround yourself with friends who make you feel safe, who share similar values, and who respect and appreciate your talents, you can become more confident, more capable, and more willing to take risks in your personal and professional life. In the crisis-intervention environment you will be helped to explore who you are and what you need from your psychological family.

Principle four: Pharmaceutical medicines are judicially used.

Thanks to the progress in biopsychiatry, medications are no longer limited to the severely mentally ill. Today, there is an assortment of medicines that will help ease your anxiety and depression. Monitored correctly by your psychiatrist, they will make your re-entry into the world an easier adjustment, as well as help you better and more quickly utilize the insights you are acquiring.

Principle five: A clear understanding that moods and behavior are being dictated by the crisis is stressed. A man suffering depression as a side effect of his blood pressure medicine looks at his family with distaste. He hates his home and his life, and he sees no way out. But as soon as the medication is stopped, his depression ends. He once again views his family with love and his life with hope. A woman who despises her stress-filled job comes home and views her personal life with the same jaundiced eye. She feels hopeless and helpless, until she quits her job and finds a more satisfying position in another firm. Suddenly everything is looking up. You too will learn to see how much biological, social, and psychological factors color your trauma—and permeate your aftershock symptoms.

Principle six: Time is needed to accept and integrate the crisis into your life. Life is not and never will be exactly what we want—or what we think we want or what we expect. We need time to rally our inner resources before we can deal realistically with the trauma. In Chapter Four, we saw how reality must sometimes be dealt out in small time-proportioned doses to desensitize the shock of the trauma. A woman who suddenly lost her husband is not ready to cope. She must go through the entire painful grieving process before the reality of her loss is accepted. In fact, studies have shown that male heart attack victims with attitudes expressed in such terms as "Hey, this isn't going to be the one to get me!" fare better than victims who are immediately besieged with the anxious, fearful realities of death. On the other hand, long-lasting denial is not good either. Witness the woman who refused to believe she had breast cancer—and didn't go to a doctor until it was too late. Crisis-intervention therapy modulates the denial/acceptance cycle, helping you find your own timetable for acceptance.

Principle Seven. Crisis-intervention therapy promotes wiser and worldlier attitudes. Life is not fair. No matter what you do, surprises—the good, the bad, and the ugly—will come your way. But if you understand that all of us are in this together, that tomorrow will be someone else's turn, you can better accept what has happened. You will realize that this pain isn't yours alone. You are not marked. You are a member of the club called humanity—with a roster that includes the famous and the infamous, the successful and the hungry, and the strong and the weak. Your crisis-intervention therapist should help you see the larger picture by revealing much of himself or herself, by showing you that no one, not even your therapist, is immune to the twists of fate.

Principle Eight. The crisis is seen as a family problem. For a more rapid recovery, your family—whether psychological or biological—must be involved. Their lives, too, have been affected by the pain of your aftershock. By enlisting your family's support and understanding, you can continue to flourish outside the therapist's office. But timing is critical; a family must be rallied with sensitivity. They too might be suffering from an aftershock that was triggered by your trauma. They might be denying your pain. They might see your problem as yours alone and not their responsibility. A good crisis-intervention therapist will solicit their help without creating a defensive atmosphere by

1. **Not coming out at the onset of your therapy and saying your pain is a family affair**
2. **Asking your family only for help not for their own therapeutic sessions**
3. **Giving them a chance to vent their own anger, dismay, and confusion**

Everyone is ambivalent. Your family's positive feelings and willingness to understand and help you do exist. With the right introduction and guidance, those attitudes can come out and be expressed in invaluable ways.

Principle Nine. Crisis therapy needs a responsive patient. Everyone is unique, and what works for you doesn't necessarily work for everyone. All of us have the potential for growth inside us, but some of us are better able to capitalize on the insights we have gained in the intensive atmosphere of crisis therapy. One woman might learn to see her traumatic divorce as a way to explore other values and other lifestyles. Another might flee from her insights, refusing to get involved with anyone again.

Principle Ten. Crisis therapy is designed for you to reestablish control over your own life. A recently divorced man in the throes of aftershock had been enraged at his ex-wife. He blamed her for everything, from not going to the theater frequently enough to gaining weight. Through his crisis-intervention therapy, he came to see that he had been in control of the situation all the time. He could have gone to the theater without his wife; he could have refused to eat fattening meals. Your crisis is an opportunity, a chance to explore your options, and to determine what you want and move toward it. You can decide your own destiny. As Rabbi Hillel once so wisely put it: "If I am not for myself, who will be for me? But if I am only for myself, then who am I? If not now, when?"

Principle Eleven. Existential themes are explored. If a therapist can help you discover a reason to live, you will find the *way* to live. If people have a terminal disease, why would they want to go on living now? Perhaps it's the chance to write the book they always wanted to write. Perhaps it's to see the birth of their new grandchild. Whatever it is, there is a reason. It's just a matter of finding it.

Principle Twelve. A comprehensive medical and social history is always taken. Your personal history not only helps your therapist determine his or her diagnosis and plan of action, it can help you understand your strengths and your vulnerabilities. A history of depression can make you more susceptible to aftershock symptoms. A series of losses early in life might make a current loss even harder to bear. Further, a comprehensive history can also help you and your therapist see

✒ The context of your life outside the confines of your trauma
✒ Your modus operandi in selecting friends, careers, and lifestyles
✒ Possible drug and alcohol abuse in an attempt to mask your pain
✒ The roles genes, illness, and past behavior play in determining your moods and your physical health

A comprehensive history brings your goals within reach faster and more accurately.

Principle Thirteen. Crisis therapy recognizes your individuality. There is never one word, one line, that is appropriate for everyone. We all are unique; we all have different ways of coping; we all have different responses to therapy. A former patient of mine and of Dr. Garfinkel illustrated the truth behind this principle. This woman, whom I call Sally, refused to see her child's suicide as anything but her fault, even when we pointed out to her that the child's father also committed suicide and that he and their daughter were suffering from schizophrenia. It was their schizophrenia and not Sally that caused their deaths. Rather than relieve her anxiety, these facts upset her even more. If she stopped taking the blame, Sally reasoned, it would mean that her other children were in danger as well because of their genes, and she couldn't live with that. In this case, trying to convince Sally that she was not at fault would have done more harm. A good crisis-intervention therapist will learn from you how much support or denial you need to get better; he or she will learn the right words of help from you.

Principle Fourteen. Reality must be confronted. We cannot bring back the dead. We cannot make a new family disappear. We cannot change the past. To adapt to a new world view, you must see reality, understand it, and accept it—at your own pace.

Principle Fifteen. Options and their limits are explored. The serenity prayer of Alcoholics Anonymous goes like this: "Lord, give me the serenity to accept what I cannot change. The courage to change what I can. And the wisdom to know the difference." Truer words were never uttered. It would be wonderful to think that the sky's the limit— at any time, in any place. But choices are not infinite. If you have no money, you can't buy your dream house tomorrow. If you are infertile, you can't get pregnant. If you are pushing fifty, you can't go back to your teens. Your options depend largely on your age, your sex, your financial stability, your health, and your social circumstances.

Your options are out there. They just have limits.

Unfortunately, when you are in the throes of aftershock, you can't see *any* options—realistic or otherwise. A crisis-intervention therapist will help you discover your real options, long-term and short. He or she will help you find the courage to make the right choices and the wisdom to know when the time is right to decide.

Principle Sixteen. The trauma is normalized. Think of it as a "reality check," an affirmation of what has happened to you within your community and your social sphere. In order to reduce your trauma's impact, it is important for others to know and accept what has happened. A man who tells a colleague about his depression will find, more times than not, that his colleague also has had his own share of suicidal thoughts. By talking about your trauma, you will gain valuable support and empathy. Suddenly and with relief you will realize that you are not as badly off as you had thought.

But spreading your news must be done with delicacy. Your therapist should help you find ways to discuss your problems and people to discuss them with. If this is done right, your social supports will be enhanced, not diminished. If it is done wrong, then, as filmmaker Frederico Fellini said, "The more sincere you are and the more you are without shame and convention, the more you expose yourself to criticism."

Principle Seventeen. Crisis therapy broadens your base of confidentiality. The goal of crisis-intervention therapy is to rapidly resolve the trauma that set off your aftershock and put it to rest. In many cases this means enlisting the aid of any "significant others" who deal with you on a daily basis. If a young teenaged girl is suicidal after losing her father, a crisis-intervention therapist might confide in her teachers to gain insight into her behavior, to alert them to any potentially dangerous signs, and to elicit more social support for the girl in her day-to-day environment.

Principle Eighteen. The focus of crisis-intervention therapy is on the present. More traditional forms of therapy search into the past for the roots of current neurotic behavior. A crisis-intervention therapist, on the other hand, is only interested in that piece of the past that has a direct bearing on your traumatic aftershock. Other than these triggers, your therapist focuses on your situation today. You don't have to go all the way back to your nasty grade-school teacher for crisis therapy to work.

Principle Nineteen. Crisis-intervention therapy uses more than one therapeutic tool. Individual psychotherapy. Group therapy. Support groups. Family therapy. Behavioral psychology. Stress management. Nutrition education. Couples therapy. Hypnosis. Biopsychiatry. Biofeedback. Massage. A crisis intervention therapist will use all the resources available to get you better fast.

Principle Twenty. Self-esteem is maintained at all times. More orthodox therapies encourage a power balance between the parent/ teacher therapist and the child/student patient. But crisis-intervention therapy is more concerned with equality, to show an aftershock victim that he or she is not alone and is not less of a person for having been dealt a traumatic blow. Yes, today your therapist is helping you grow, but tomorrow the situation could be reversed. As Rainer Maria Rilke wrote in *Letters to a Young Poet*, "Do not believe that he who seeks to comfort you lives untroubled among the simple and quiet words that sometimes do you good. His life has much difficulty and sadness . . . were it otherwise he would have never have been able to find those words."

In the next two chapters, I will be going over the wide range of therapies available today in crisis intervention. The first chapter will introduce you to the variety of medications that can ease your aftershock symptoms in conjunction with the therapies outlined in the second chapter. Read each entry. Think about them. And remember, above all, you are not alone. Help is at hand. You can be set free.

G O O D   N E W S
A B O U T   M E D I C I N E

THEIR NAMES SOUND LIKE DOUBLETALK FROM A Latin Cheshire cat. They are multisyllable, multiparticle chemicals that most laymen can barely pronounce. They are the "anti" drugs of a new generation: antianxiety, antipsychotic, antidepressant, antimanic, that may be helpful in treating the symptoms of aftershock (such as anxiety) or the conditions that may either be caused by or associated with aftershock. And they are changing the scope and the possibilities of psychiatry in ways that Freud and his peers would never even have dreamed was possible.

In the past three decades, the link between body and mind has become progressively better understood. From the neurotransmitters that carry message impulses through the brain to the actual brain sections that carry out the tasks, biopsychiatry has changed our views of anxiety, depression, and irrational behavior for good. Its sister science, psychopharmacology, has made inroads into the study of mood-altering

161

drugs, helping to create safer, more predictable, and better working medicines that, in conjunction with psychotherapy, bring new promise for the 1980s.

MYTH: People who take medication for psychological problems belong in a hospital.
FACT: One out of every ten adults in America today takes a mild tranquilizer at least once a year.
MYTH: Pain relievers are the number-one category of prescribed medications in America.
FACT: More prescriptions are dispensed for insomnia and anxiety than for any other condition.
MYTH: Medications, especially psychiatric medications, are not safe.
FACT: All medications, especially the psychiatric medications, are extremely safe when administered by a competent physician, and when the patient follows his or her doctor's advice.
MYTH: When people get depressed, all they have to do is talk to someone about it. They will get over it.
FACT: Depression, when not caught in its early stages, will frequently get progressively worse. Medicine, given in conjunction with psychotherapy, helps an estimated 70 percent of all despondent persons.

Now more than ever, we need a cure for the effects produced by our many pressure points. Now more than ever, we need hope. Now, thanks to the new medicines of the mind, we have both.

IT'S ALL IN THE MIND

Before people can gain control of the effects of their traumatic event, they must gain control of their emotions. Medications, properly administered, can help them do just that.

As we have seen in Chapter Ten, medications are a crucial element of crisis-intervention therapy. If a man is suicidal, he needs relief —fast. If a woman is suffering from such severe anxiety she can't set foot outside her door, she needs to feel less threatened—fast. If a teenager is showing fits of violence in the classroom, he needs his emotions balanced—fast. Therapy alone is time consuming. People need to go out of their house, to earn a living, to communicate with their family, even as therapy progresses.

Pharmaceuticals can help show the suicidal man that all is not bleak. They can help to free the woman from her self-imposed prison. They can steady the teenager and calm his erratic violence. They can make all the difference between functioning in the real world or not.

The view of life people in the throes of aftershock see is colored by their trauma. It is difficult to see beyond the pain. But if the anxieties or the depressions or the panicky feelings can be eased, victims will become more open to the insights they gain in their therapist's office. Without the cloud of their debilitating aftershock symptoms, they will be more motivated and better able to help themselves move toward health.

Without pharmaceuticals, aftershock sufferers will often remain in pain much longer, continually bombarded by stimuli that bring back the trauma loud and clear. Most will not be able to think clearly. And clear thinking is necessary to ultimately desensitize the trauma, to put it in its rightful time and place, to get on with life.

But drugs alone are not a panacea. They need to be administered by an experienced and competent psychiatrist, and in order for their benefits to continue, they must be used in combination with regular therapy.

DRUG TALK

Becky had the attitude, "live and let live." She had always managed to take things in stride, and recently as a marketing manager of a large textile firm, she had managed to take care of both her new baby and her high-pressure job with flair. When she was at home, she didn't think about the office; when she was in the office, she delegated the work so well that she was able to fit in regular exercise and vacations twice a year. But all that changed when her husband came home and asked for a divorce. It was as if the ground had opened up and plunged Becky down into a terrifying other world. She could no longer stay organized; she found herself running ragged and, when she wasn't crying late into the night, she was having terrible nightmares.

Things went from bad to worse. The day she was panic-stricken at the thought of going to the office and seeing people she knew she needed help.

Becky was put on an antianxiety medication, but not before her psychiatrist determined that pharmaceutical therapy was the right approach for her. In accordance with standard procedure, the psychiatrist considered the following factors:

⚡ The symptoms had lasted for over four weeks.

⚡ The cause of her anxiety was not a physical one.

⚡ There were no signs of liver disease, ulcers, or circulatory problems.

⚡ Pregnancy was not an issue.

⚡ Alcohol would not be consumed.

⚡ No other medication would interact adversely with the antianxiety medication.

⚡ Instructions, explanations, and possible side effects were completely understood by Becky.

Throughout Becky's drug therapy, her blood levels were monitored to make sure she was getting the right amount of medicine into her bloodstream. Age, other medications, and conditions could all adversely affect the drug level in her system. If she had been pregnant, the risks to her unborn baby could be severe. And alcohol consumption could produce severe side effects—possibly resulting in death.

Coffee and cigarette smoking, on the other hand, both *decrease* the drug's effectiveness level. If Becky, both a light coffee drinker and a nonsmoker, were to increase or acquire these respective habits during her therapy, the drug might not have any effect at all—and her anxiety would return.

Becky's psychiatrist also periodically checked to make sure she was taking her medication properly. A major reason why people fail to benefit from medication is that they frequently stop taking it or do not take the recommended dosage. In fact, noncompliance in drug therapy can range from 30 percent to 60 percent, depending on the psychological problem and the treatment schedule.

But compliance can make all the difference between making drug therapy a success or a time-wasting failure. Frequently, when patients feel better under drug therapy, they mistakenly think that they are cured and no longer need the medication. Unfortunately the symptoms usually return when the medication stops, sometimes even more severely than before. Other individuals, after experiencing a side effect such as nausea or headaches, decide without informing their doctor to stop taking the medication. Or they may have difficulty adhering to their dosing schedule. To compound the problem, these patients frequently neglect later to inform their psychiatrists that they stopped taking the drug; they simply report that the medication doesn't work, making the process of finding the best medicine for them even more difficult.

Whatever the reason, a good psychiatrist will try to anticipate the possibility of a patient's noncompliance. An irresponsible patient, or one whose ability to function is limited by aftershock, may find a dosing schedule of two pills every four hours difficult to maintain; in this case a medication with a once-a-day dose would prove the better choice.

The following box includes some of the questions a psychiatrist might ask to gauge a patient's ability to comply with the medication. In

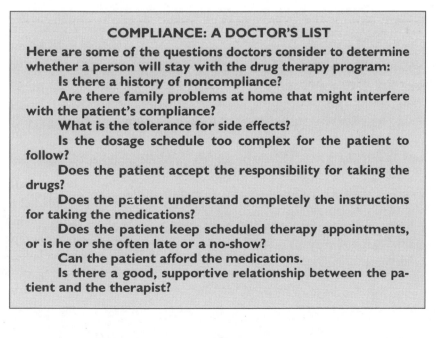

COMPLIANCE: A DOCTOR'S LIST

Here are some of the questions doctors consider to determine whether a person will stay with the drug therapy program:

Is there a history of noncompliance?

Are there family problems at home that might interfere with the patient's compliance?

What is the tolerance for side effects?

Is the dosage schedule too complex for the patient to follow?

Does the patient accept the responsibility for taking the drugs?

Does the patient understand completely the instructions for taking the medications?

Does the patient keep scheduled therapy appointments, or is he or she often late or a no-show?

Can the patient afford the medications.

Is there a good, supportive relationship between the patient and the therapist?

many cases, a psychiatrist should monitor the patient's blood levels to insure that the patient is getting the most effective dose.

Pharmacology and biopsychiatry are sciences. Like all sciences, they are not exact. Mathematics solves one equation only to find infinite possibilities in its answer. Astronomy discovers one star only to find an entire galaxy behind it. Medicine heralds one breakthrough cure only to find it can be improved. The possibilities are always there; pharmaceuticals create new variables even as progress is being made. Metabolism, age, symptoms, severity of side effects, success rate, personal habits, physical health—all have their influence on which drug a person should take, the dosage, length of treatment, and how well it works.

It is these variables that make it crucial for drug therapy to be supervised by a psychiatrist. You should never attempt to medicate yourself. The very best that could happen is no effect at all. The very worst is grave harm to both your mental and physical state.

ALCOHOL: THE SELF-MEDICATION PUBLIC ENEMY NUMBER ONE

"Drowning your sorrows in alcohol"—Unfortunately, these words are more to the point than you might think. Studies have shown that alcohol does indeed relieve anxiety, but only on a short-term basis. The more you drink, the less effective drinking becomes in this respect.

Successful aftershock treatment depends, as we have seen in Chapter Ten, on how well you integrate the trauma into your new view of the world: understanding it, accepting it, and putting it into its proper context. When you drink, you might reexperience the crisis, venting your anger and your pain, but it is never integrated into your world view. Reliving your trauma in an alcoholic state is superficial and doomed to failure. You never truly understand and accept it. The next morning, instead of a catharsis, instead of overcoming your aftershock, you have a hangover.

Further, drinking can lead to alcohol abuse, which only adds another symptom to your aftershock list. Drowning, after all, is but another form of death.

MEDICINE SHOW

Psychopharmacology is researching new drugs even as I write. The list can go on and on and provide material for another book. But to help you through the maze of drug therapy, I've broken down the different types of pills into five categories: antianxiety drugs or mild tranquilizers, antidepressants, antimanics, antiadrenal blockers, and antipsychotics or major tranquilizers. For each category, you will find *brief* descriptions of what the drugs are used for, their history, their characteristics, some of their potential side effects and withdrawal symptoms, and their most common names.

By no means is this information intended to replace the proper medical care and supervision of a physician; there is simply no substitute for the experience and information a doctor can provide. It is extremely important that when taking any medication you follow your doctor's directions. If you experience any unusual symptoms or side effects while taking a medication, contact your doctor immediately.

This information is provided solely to help you reach a basic understanding of the types of drugs that may be used in the treatment of aftershock. With this understanding, and most important with the supervision of a competent physician, you can begin to find a way back from aftershock. Let us start.

ANTIANXIETY DRUGS OR MILD TRANQUILIZERS

These are the most common mood-altering drugs. With the exception of barbiturates, they are also among the safest. Prominent among antianxiety drugs are the benzodiazepines (just think of "BZ" for short). They are considered the drugs of first choice in the treatment of anxiety, and are very effective. A list of these drugs includes brands that are almost household names: Xanax, Valium, and Librium.

I. The BZs (Benzodiazepines)

Common brand names include: Xanax, Valium, Librium, Ativan, Serox, Tranxene, and Dalmane.
Use: Primarily to treat anxiety; may also be used for insomnia, panic attacks, alcohol withdrawal, and obsessive/compulsive behavior.
History: Though this group was discovered in the 1930s, it was not until

the 1950s, when a group of research monkeys became noticeably calmer from a dose of a BZ compound, that scientists found it of therapeutic value. As soon as they were deemed safe for humans, BZs took the market by storm.

Characteristics: Work before an anxiety attack begins; stop anticipation of a fearful event rather than halt the attack in progress. Can become habit forming. Alcohol should always be avoided when taking BZs. Because anxiety, as Freud said, is a signal that something is wrong, these medications can mask real problems; they treat the symptoms rather than the disease. Usually best taken in conjunction with therapy.

Possible side effects include: drowsiness, impairment of both coordination and intellectual functioning.

Withdrawal: Includes restlessness, depression, headaches, nausea, lack of focus, and irritability. Can be severe; best to taper off dosage under doctor's supervision.

A new antianxiety agent, buspirone (brand name BuSpar) is not classified as a benzodiazepine. Reportedly, this medication does not have the addictive properties of the BZs.

2. Barbiturates

Common brand names include: Amytal, Mebaral, and Nembutal.

Use: In lower doses to treat anxiety; in higher doses to treat insomnia.

History: Known for over 100 years; Used initially to treat epileptics; Became a popular drug for insomnia until the BZs were discovered to be safer and less habit forming.

Characteristics: Can lead to addiction. Best used in hospitals where patients can be watched for potential overdose; Can be fatal if mixed with alcohol.

Possible side effects include: Extreme drowsiness, difficult breathing, and skin rash.

Withdrawal: Severe; similar to alcohol withdrawal.

ANTIDEPRESSANTS

The most common antidepressants, called tricyclic antidepressants or TCAs for short, are the first line of treatment for depression when drug therapy is indicated. The good news is that they work in 60 percent to 85 percent of the cases.

The bad news is they need time to take effect. Patients usually need two to four weeks before they can get relief. And sometimes patients cannot tolerate their side effects.

The other major class of drugs used against depression includes the monoamine oxidase (MAO) inhibitors.

Together, these drugs have changed the face of depression therapy forever. Quite simply they fight depression in two different ways. The MAO inhibitors block the action of an enyzme called monamine oxidase, or MAO, that is thought to be responsible for breaking down the neurotransmitters that regulate a person's emotional state. MAO inhibitors act to correct the unbalanced emotional state that characterizes depression. The tricyclics (TCAs) are newer and have largely replaced the MAO inhibitors as the drug of choice. They, too, increase the brain's level of neurotransmitters but via a different route. Their side effects are fewer and they have a higher proven success rate.

Whichever drug your psychiatrist prescribes, follow his or her instructions explicitly. Ask any questions you might have. And above all be patient. Real relief from your debilitating depression may only be a few weeks away.

2. TCAs

Common brand names include: Elavil, Tofranil, Pamelor, Sinequan, Arentyl, Anafronil, and Norpramin.

Use: Depression; anxiety and panic attacks; phobias including agoraphobia (fear of public places).

History: TCAs are short for tricyclics, named for their three-ring molecular composition. Newer, safer, and more effective than the MAO inhibitors, these drugs have become the most popular in antidepressant drug therapy. In one study of depressed war veterans suffering from aftershock, 82 percent improved with TCA therapy.

Possible side effects include: Dry mouth, blurry vision, constipation, sleepiness, rapid pulse, and difficult urination.

Withdrawal: Dosage should be gradually reduced under a doctor's supervision.

I. MAO Inhibitors

Common brand names include: Marplan, Nardil, and Parnate.

Use: Depression, anxiety, nightmares, hallucinations, daytime flashbacks.

History: The first of the popular antidepressant drugs; a breakthrough in biopsychiatry.

Characteristics: Effective in aiding aftershock victims to relieve trauma so that the event can be more readily integrated; used for depressions that do not respond to other therapy, or when patient cannot tolerate other medication. Dietary restrictions and potential for severe side effects limit their use.

Patients *must* avoid fermented food like beer, wine, and cheese and medications such as amphetamines and many over-the-counter cough, cold, and hay fever products, because the combination can cause extreme high blood pressure that can be fatal. (Contact your doctor or pharmacist for a complete list of foods and drugs that must be avoided.)

Possible side effects include: Headache, nausea, vomiting, rapid or irregular heartbeat, dilated pupils, stiff neck, and inability to tolerate light.

Withdrawal: Should be tapered off gradually under a doctor's supervision.

ANTIMANICS

Everyone feels bad some days, good the next. But when mood swings are abnormally high and low, they can be deadly. In the depressed state, people can become suicidal; in the manic state, they can destroy their families as they take them on a joy ride of violence and extravagant, wired, self-delusioned actions that border on the psychotic. Drugs that balance out these highs and lows are called antimanics and they are primarily used for aftershock symptoms that are violent, overly aggressive, antisocial, and out of control. In fact, one study found that eight out of fourteen PTSD victims stopped reexperiencing their traumas after being given an antimanic drug.

Lithium Carbonate

Common brand names include: Lithium, Eskolith, Lithane.

Use: A mood stabilizer for treating manic depression, and possibly for treatment of PTSD.

History: A natural mineral salt that was discovered to stop manic behavior in 70 percent of all cases.

Characteristics: Most manic-depressives need high levels to maintain emotional equilibrium; appears to reduce the reexperiencing of the trauma in aftershock victims.

Possible side effects include: Drowsiness, restlessness, confusion, hallucinations, headache, nausea, vomiting, diarrhea, and rash.

Withdrawal: Only under the supervision of a physician.

ANTIADRENAL BLOCKERS

The hunter hones in on his prey. As he unleashes his arrow, his body unleashes adrenaline, preparing him for a fight or a fast flight. As I discussed in Chapter Four, this fight-or-flight phenomenon occurs whenever we have a potentially stressful stimulus. Unfortunately, in most cases we can't take a fighter's stance—or run away from home. But the adrenaline surge continues, with no place to go. This situation is particularly common in aftershock victims who continue to play back their traumas. Stimuli in their environment keep their adrenaline flowing; their adrenaline keeps them on the lookout for stimuli.

That is where these blockers come in. They effectively block our automatic responses to stimuli, so that the sudden noise in the night is not a replay of the prowler, the dripping faucet is not the flood, the man walking down the street is not our dead spouse.

There are two kinds of blockers; both work in similar ways. One is the alpha adrenergic agonist and the other is the beta blocker. Let's look at them:

I. Alpha adrenergic agonist

Common brand names include: Catapres, Minipress.

Use: Primarily in the treatment of high blood pressure, but may also be used for anxiety and to lessen the fear of trauma recurring.

History: Since the physical symptoms of anxiety often include rapid heartbeat, and elevated blood pressure, researchers examined whether medications that reduced these symptoms might also lower anxiety. In fact, these drugs were found to have anxiety-mitigating effects.

Characteristics: Following their administration, a patient may notice a decrease in anxiety attacks or violent outbursts, intrusive flashbacks, nightmares, or startled responses.

Possible side effects include: Dry mouth, drowsiness, constipation, dizziness, headache, and fatigue.

Withdrawal: Usually a gradual reduction in dosage under doctor's supervision is best.

2. Beta blocker (BBs)

Common brand names include: Inderal, Corgard, Lopressor, Tenormin.
Use: Primarily in the treatment of high blood pressure and heart disease; BBs may also be used to treat anxiety; stage fright.
History: Same as for alpha adrenergic agonist.
How it works: Similar to alpha adrenergic agonist but more selective; works on the peripheral nervous system.
Characteristics: Dosage is based on heartbeat; resting pulse must be decreased by eight or more beats; patients must take their pulse every day to monitor; does not work on phobic aftershock symptoms.
Possible side effects include: Sleeplessness, sexual impotency, asthma, nausea, and fatigue.
Withdrawal: Should be reduced gradually, under doctor's supervision.

ANTIPSYCHOTICS OR MAJOR TRANQUILIZERS

These are the drugs of last resort. Sometimes called neuroleptics, sometimes major tranquilizers, they are used for major psychotic episodes, for aftershock victims who cannot tell if a hallucinatory flashback is real or not, who are wracked with delusions, and who more times than not have exacerbated their condition with drugs or alcohol. They produce a sense of calm—but at a price. Most prominent among the antipsychotics are a class of drugs called phenothiazines.

Phenothiazines

Common brand names include: Thorazine, Serentil, Mellaril, Trilafon, Prolixin, and Stelazine.
Use: Primarily for schizophrenia and other psychotic conditions; may also be used to reduce extreme agitation and restlessness.
History: Chlorpramize (the generic or chemical name for Thorazine) was first used by veterinarians to rid animals of parasites. Later, in the 1950s, Thorazine was used to prepare patients for surgery. Soon researchers noted that in lower doses the drug alleviated the psychotic symptoms of schizophrenia, allowing many previously hospitalized patients to lead normal lives outside of institutions.
Characteristics: Bring calmness while relieving hallucinations, and de-

lusions. The potential for developing a serious side effect called tardive dyskinesia (a condition characterized by sudden tics or jerks of the face, tongue, or body) severely restricts the use of these drugs. Long-term use (for one year or more) of antipsychotic medications may result in 10 percent to 20 percent of the patients developing tardive dyskinesia.

Possible side effects include: Constipation, dry mouth, blurry vision, rigid muscles or tremors; rapid heartbeat, difficult urination, muscle spasms, and twitching.

Withdrawal: Should be withdrawn gradually and under the supervision of a physician.

Other major tranquilizers include thiothixene (Navane), haloperidol (Haldol), and clozapine (Clozaril).

These are just a few of the medicines of the mind in very broad terms. Once again, this listing is meant solely as an introduction to the brave new worlds of psychiatry. Do not attempt to medicate yourself or anyone else. By all means rely on a competent doctor for the most effective drug therapy.

QUESTIONS, ANYONE?

The more we learn, the less we know. I hope that this chapter both answered some of your questions about drug therapy and prompted new ones.

Before we go on, take a look at these commonly asked questions about drug therapy and their answers. They can help clarify what you have learned—and what you want to know.

Q. I've been diagnosed as depressed. My doctor gave me both an antidepressant and an antianxiety pill. Why?

A: Sometimes you can become anxious at the fact that you are depressed. Your doctor may feel that the antianxiety pill will help to relieve the stress.

Q: What's the difference between Valium and Xanax?

A: The difference between these drugs concerns primarily the length of time they take to achieve their effects. Valium takes a longer time to go through your bloodstream. If you are chronically anxious or suffering from insomnia, Valium is your best bet. Because Xanax, on the other hand, is short lived, it is better for spurts of panic. This way you won't become lethargic after the situation that has panicked you has passed. In addition, Xanax may prove to be an effective treatment for other anxiety disorders and depression.

Q: What's the difference between unipolar and bipolar depressions?

A: Briefly, unipolar depressions are not accompanied by periods of mania (or euphoria); bipolar depressions are seen in people who are also, at times, manic.

Q: The drug I'm taking doesn't seem to do anything for me. What should I do?

A: First of all, be sure to discuss the situation with your psychiatrist. Antidepressants may need several weeks before they begin to take effect. But if you see no sign of improvement for many weeks, then your doctor should consider adjusting your dosage or using a different drug. People are as varied as the different medicines available. What works for one doesn't necessarily work for another. Often finding the best drug—and its dosage—is a case of trial and error until the right match is found.

Q: I just got a prescription for an antianxiety pill. How long must I take it?

A: That's a question for your psychiatrist. Only he or she is monitoring your blood level and completely understands your condition. On the average, 50 percent of the people taking antianxiety pills stop after six weeks. But studies show that within no more than twelve months, their symptoms come back. So in the long run, it may be best to opt for longer-term treatment to insure that your anxiety has completely disappeared.

These then are the medicines of the mind, the drugs that combined with proper therapy can help to free you from your aftershock prison. In the next chapter, I will be going over the various therapies that work in crisis situations. Join me. Growth, mental health, and peace of mind are waiting.

THERAPY THAT REALLY WORKS

Men are disturbed not by things,
but by the views they take of them.
—Epictetus, Greek Philosopher

WE CANNOT CHANGE THE STRESSFUL LIFE EVENTS that affect us. But we can change the *way* they affect us. We have seen the role that pharmaceuticals play in this process. Now we will turn to psychology and look at the therapies available today for aftershock—therapies that really work.

One person out of every twenty goes into therapy each year. In thirty-nine years, the number of clinical psychology programs in the United States has more than tripled: from twenty-nine in 1947 to one hundred and forty-three in 1986. More and more, therapy is becoming an accepted—and necessary—component of modern life.

From strict Freudian analysis to support self-help groups, there are as many approaches to mental health as there are therapists. And no one therapy is absolute. What will work for you might not work for someone else.

As we saw in Chapter Eleven, biopsychiatry is a science, using the advances made in neurological medicine to create mood-altering pharmaceuticals and repair dysfunctioning brain passageways. Psychotherapy is more of an art; self-destructive thoughts and patterns are interpreted by a therapist and discussed. The more skilled the therapist, the better the insights. The better the insights, the better—and faster—your mental growth. Combined, biological and psychological treatment can assure complete recovery and continued health. Together, they can help you push through your pain for good.

When asked why he was in therapy for over fifteen years, Woody Allen's character in *Annie Hall* said "I'm going to give it one more year. . . . then I'm going to Lourdes." Hopefully, this chapter will help you circumvent those fifteen years of searching and get it right the first time.

A GOOD FIT

In his book *The Technique of Psychotherapy* (Grune & Stratton, 1977), Lewis Wolberg defined three goals of psychotherapy:

1 **Removing, modifying, or retarding existing symptoms**
2 **Mediating disturbed patterns of behavior**
3 **Promoting positive personality growth and development**

Training varies with the therapist. Psychiatrists must go through medical school, internship, and residency programs. Only they can dispense prescription drugs. Psychotherapists run the range from Doctorates in Philosophy to Master Degrees in psychology. There are also certified social workers and psychiatric nurses who are licensed to practice psychotherapy. In addition therapists must go through an extensive training program if they plan to specialize in, say, Freudian, Jungian, or behavioral psychology.

It is this training and experience that separates a therapist from a friend. Therapists are skilled in the dynamics and techniques of treating emotional problems; they look at what is not being said as much as what is. They are presumably objective, keeping their own values to themselves. They too have been through analysis, and by setting up a payment schedule they keep your relationship formal.

But more than any other factor, it is the relationship you have with your therapist that will make the process a success—or a failure. It is crucial that you can feel comfortable with him or her; you must feel a sense of consistency and safety. You must feel an emotional rapport so that when the air becomes tense, you will continue to be motivated. This is why first visits are usually set up as "interviews" so both you and your therapist can decide if you can work together and develop a fruitful trust.

In Chapter Ten, I discussed the fact that crisis intervention uses any and all therapies available to promote fast healing and growth. Now, one by one, I will deal with those therapies and the way they help cure aftershock's pain.

WHAT DID YOU MEAN BY THAT? OR INDIVIDUAL PSYCHOTHERAPY

Say psychotherapy and people will almost automatically think of Sigmund Freud. A neurologist by profession, he began his work on the human psyche at the end of the nineteenth century. Today his conceptions of the id, superego, and ego, his theories on defense mechanisms, and his ideas on the stages of childhood development are familiar to anyone who has taken Psychology 101. Aside from Marx and Einstein, no one has influenced twentieth century civilization more than Freud.

The core of his "psychodynamic theory" was his belief that behavior is governed by deep, unconscious motives that were formed in early childhood. If a person is malfunctioning in the present, these motives must be unearthed and understood. And the process of "making the unconscious, conscious" is called psychoanalysis.

We all know the cliche of the patient, lying on the couch, spewing out his thoughts to the silent therapist who sits out of view writing notes. The room we conjure up is paneled; a soft lamp illuminates the oriental carpeting and the primitive art. It is womb-like, all the better to beckon the unconscious mind.

Like most cliches, this one is based on truth. Patients do lie on couches—once a day, several times a week and more times than not, for many years. Through free association (where the patient talks about anything that comes to mind), dream interpretation (where the symbols of unconscious desires are vividly portrayed), transference (where the therapist takes on the role of the patient's mother or father), and resistance (where the patient tries to stop a threatening exploration),

Freudian psychiatrists can pinpoint what they see as their patients' unconscious motivations and in turn help them understand why they act and feel the way they do. When confronted, the motivations that have been repressed and stored in the unconscious, would lose their power. A patient could then go on with his or her life, unencumbered by the guilt and anxiety of an unresolved past.

Over the years, psychoanalysis has lost its appeal. Though it gives you an intellectual understanding of your psyche, it doesn't necessarily give you the ability to act in healthier ways. It is extremely time consuming and expensive, and in today's aftershock world, there are better methods of treatment.

Freud's influence can be found in modern one-on-one therapies but not in a strict psychoanalytical sense. Today's psychotherapy involves the patient and the therapist in an active dialogue; they both sit in chairs and face each other. Patient and therapist may meet only once or twice a week; the total time consumed in therapy sessions may be less. The interpretation of your present and the people currently in your life plays as important a role as the interpretation of your past. Therapy is more eclectic; whatever helps you cope with the world and promotes understanding is used.

But even contemporary individual therapy is time consuming.

✒ It can take years for patients to develop a strong enough trust in their therapist to "open up."

✒ Threatened by the burgeoning revelation of what they believe to be their inadequacies, patients will begin to resist the treatment; they will try to hold on to their comfortable, familiar, but ultimately damaging behavior to keep a sense of self-worth.

✒ By its very psychodynamic definition, therapy is constantly being changed by the outside world. A man could discover that he has been married to the wrong woman. A woman could lose her job. A family could feel threatened by the therapy and try to sabotage it.

✒ The reasons why you are in therapy can change, until at long last the underlying anxieties come out.

✒ Even termination can be difficult and time consuming. Patients can become nervous over the prospect of leaving; they can regress. In my book with Margaret Raymond and Julian Lieb, *The*

SCHOOLS OF THOUGHT:
OTHER FORMS OF PSYCHOTHERAPY

The Humanistic-Existentialist Therapy

The Humanistic-Existentialist (H-E) therapists see the essential conflict as not being between the unconscious and conscious minds, but rather between the person's lofty view of what they would like to be (the ideal self) and their negative view of whom they really are (the self-concept). An individual with a negative self-concept produces anxiety at their inability to reach the ideal self. A *humanist* therapist blames a person's upbringing for causing this dichotomy: A child may be told that they must always be the best; while anything they do accomplish is never good enough. The anxiety that arises from this split prevents an individual from growing and blossoming as a human.

A popular variation of the humanistic approach, called *"client-centered therapy,"* was developed by Carl Rogers. According to Rogers, troubled individuals need only to be respected and understood by another person (i.e. the therapist). The goal of client-centered therapy is to "hear" what the individual is actually thinking and feeling, and then to show that the therapist understands and accepts these feelings by restating the individual's thoughts. According to this theory, the unconditional acceptance that the therapist gives improves the patient's self-concept.

Like the psychodynamic and humanistic therapists, *existentialists* are not very concerned with specific symptoms of anxiety, but focus on the intrapsychic conflict. While very similar to humanistic therapists, existentialists see the intrapsychic conflict arising not from the struggle between the self-concept and the ideal self, but rather from the struggle between the values of the individual and the forces of society that act against these values. The goal of existentialist therapy is to help the patient live "authentically," according to their values, in today's society.

Healing Alliance (W. W. Norton, 1975), we wrote of a compulsive school teacher who had been building a stone wall in his backyard. When he began, he religiously used a plumbline. Later, he no longer needed to rely on exact, rigid measurements to build his wall. At that point, he realized he didn't need to rely on his therapy either. He knew he could quit.

But time is a luxury aftershock victims can't afford. And in many cases the financial cost is more than they can handle. That is where emergency psychotherapy comes in.

Emergency One-on-one

To circumvent the long process of discovering the underlying reasons for therapy, a crisis interventionist will start with a differential diagnosis, a concise method of determining symptoms and causes. First of all, a patient can be brought into a hospital on the brink of death; quick relief is needed. Second, though the medicines for both traumatically based and neurotically based anxiety are the same, the modes of therapeutic treatments are different. People who have been suffering from anxiety their entire lives need long-term therapy to work out their problems completely. People suffering from a stressful life-changing event can get the help they need with short-term, focused therapy.

And once the traumatic root is established, a crisis-intervention therapist must make sure that therapy is even needed. A study of acute grief reactions by W. Vail Williams and Paul R. Polak found that crisis-intervention therapy could actually be harmful if it stops the normal stages of grief.

Emergency psychotherapy includes many of the principles of crisis intervention I outlined in Chapter Ten. A therapist's goal is to guide the patient through abreaction—the reexperiencing of the trauma so it can be put into its rightful time and place once and for all.

The actual process is two fold, cognitive and structural. The cognitive element deals with the subjective, underlying fears and anxieties in a patient's mind. The structural element is more pragmatic and reinforces the cognitive element with concrete situations. Here is how they work together to turn the anxiety of a crisis into growth.

A teenage boy named Jim had lost a close friend in a tragic accident. He began to withdraw from school, his other friends, and his parents. This withdrawal led to hostile behavior, especially to his parents. He became an angry and violent stranger in his home. Cognitively, the therapist helped Jim examine his values and explore what he was feeling about the trauma and how that related to the way he was acting toward his parents. Structurally, the therapist encouraged Jim's parents to take the boy out to dinner and to begin to open communications with him.

Finally, emergency psychotherapy shares a secret with all individual therapies: helping a patient face the ultimate reality of death. This fear is at the core of neurotic behavior, of any traumatic experience—and of eventual growth. We are indeed all a part of that tenacious, glorious, and complex family called man.

As psychologist Carl Rogers once said: "The task of psychotherapy is to help the person achieve, through the special relationship with a therapist, good communication within himself. Once this is achieved, he can communicate more freely and effectively with others. We may then say that psychotherapy is good communication within and between men. Good communication, free communication, with and between men, is always therapeutic."

ACTIONS SPEAK LOUDER THAN WORDS—OR BEHAVIOR THERAPY

Whereas psychotherapy follows Freud's tenet that all behavior stems from unconscious motives, behaviorists believe that the motives lie very close to the surface indeed that the behavior itself holds the answers.

The birth of behaviorism came in the early part of the century with Pavlov's famous salivating dogs. Sounding an alarm bell at the same time he offered them food, he eventually trained them to salivate at the sound of the bell alone, proving that responses to stimuli could be learned, that we can be conditioned to respond in a certain way.

Others came along: Watson, who believed that all emotions were conditioned responses to certain stimuli; Thorndike, who explored how we learn to respond to different stimuli; Skinner, who discovered that responses could be reinforced by rewards or changed by punishment.

Behaviorism today has much appeal. It is a fast, focused therapy that deals entirely in the present. A behavior therapist is not interested in your past. He or she is concerned with your actions today, not with your internal motivations. He or she takes your actions at face value and tries to change them for the better.

Sometimes a behavior therapist will draw up a contract, explaining that you will be given a reward when you behave in a certain way. For example, a woman trying to diet might receive a reward after she lost ten pounds.

Sometimes the therapist will use stimulus control so that you respond to one cue and one cue only. If you have had trouble sleeping, you are taught to use your bed for sleeping only, not reading, watching television, or talking on the phone.

Another technique involves role modeling. If you see your therapist, a person you admire, acting a certain way, you will begin to imitate him or her. If you see that person boarding a plane without fear, you will try to overcome your phobia for plane travel.

This world of behavior modification has vast applications for aftershock victims. Since so many stimuli in the outside world remind you of your trauma, you are conditioned to respond with the same anxiety, fear, and panic you felt when the trauma first occurred. Becky, the recently divorced woman I talked about in Chapter Eleven, kept thinking about her husband every time she heard a song on the radio; she thought about him when it rained, because it had rained the night he left her. She wanted to cry every time she saw a couple walking down the street, because they reminded her of the days long ago when she and her husband had been in love.

But if Becky could change the way she responded to these almost continuous stimuli, her aftershock would disappear and her trauma could be laid to rest. Let's look at some of the behavior therapies that have worked for aftershock symptoms.

The pain that cures

Aversion therapy has had great success with alcoholics and drug addicts. Here, electric shocks or nausea-producing drugs are given to a patient at the same time as, in the case of an alcoholic, a glass of scotch. Over time, the stimulus of the drink is given a negative connotation; the response is no longer pleasurable, and a person no longer desires a drink.

Hard shells are made

Instead of aversion therapy's method of turning a pleasurable stimulus into an awful one, systematic desensitization turns a fearful stimulus into a neutral one. We learn to develop a thick skin to the things that have always brought on panic and fear. First, a patient is taught to relax using a form of self-hypnosis (more on this later). Then, he or she writes down a personal inventory of fears, beginning with the scariest image and moving to the least anxiety-provoking one. Remember Rosemarie from Chapter Three, the woman who had developed an aftershock phobia of cockroaches after finding one in her muffin? If she went for systematic desensitization therapy, she might start her list with cockroaches crawling all over her. She would end with seeing a dead cockroach in a natural history museum. After the list has been completed, the patient, in a relaxed state, is shown slides of his or her hierarchy of fears, beginning with the mildest image and ending with the worst one. If the patient remains calm, he or she becomes desensitized to the cues that have always been terrifying. Rosemarie would find that the sense of calm she felt when she saw the images in her therapist's office carried through to real life. She would be able to eat in a restaurant without fear; she would stop looking compulsively for cockroaches in her apartment.

Thinking is believing

Finally there is cognitive therapy, a branch of behaviorism based on the belief that it is our thoughts that govern our behavior. Cognitive therapists do not share the traditional behaviorist's view that actions can be changed by modifying a stimulus. Rather they feel that if we change the way we think, we can change the way we act, regardless of the outside stimulus. It is our thoughts that control how we will respond to cues—in a positive manner or in a self-destructive one.

Through anywhere from twelve to twenty weeks, a cognitive therapist works closely with a patient, pinpointing where faulty reasoning has made the patient depressed, guilty, or anxious. It is an intense, active therapy; you are encouraged to do homework assignments that help you see logically where your thinking has led you astray. Someone who feels guilty all the time might be asked to write down the times of day he or she felt guilty, and why. A perfectionist who constantly feels the pressure of obligation might be asked to clock in every time the word "should" enters his or her mind. Someone who feels tremendous anxiety whenever it is time to go to a business meeting might be asked to write down the percentage of "hard work" it would take to go into the meeting plus the percentage of positive feeling that would be felt after it was over. Then, once the meeting was actually over, he or she would write down the actual hard work percentage—which would al-

183

ways be much lower than what was envisioned. And the percentage of positive energy from completing the dreaded task would always be much higher!

Logically and systematically a cognitive therapist will show you where you have been using faulty reasoning—from de-emphasizing the positive and black-and-white "all or nothing" attitudes to jumping to conclusions and overgeneralizing—and help you see how rational thinking can make you immediately feel better about yourself.

Though cognitive therapy can help people with all sorts of problem behavior, its main inroads have been into depression and that's where its use as an aftershock therapy tool is invaluable.

Dr. Aaron T. Beck, the founder of cognitive therapy, discovered that depressed people have an inherent negative personality schema—where every facet of their lives is seen in a negative light. A trauma can set this schema into action, reinforcing and strengthening this negative outlook. The trauma's aftermath, with its feelings of hopelessness and dependency, continues to build up depressed, negative thoughts.

Using many of the techniques I have outlined above, the therapist brings the depressed person to see how life really isn't as negative or as bleak as he or she had thought.

In their excellent book, *Abnormal Psychology: Current Perspectives*, fifth edition (Random House, 1988), Richard Bootzin and Joan Ross Acocella present a list of cognitive retraining assignments similar to the following list. (Please note that Bootzin and Acocella reprinted this list from a paper presented by R. C. Bedrosian and A. T. Beck.)

Here is an example of a cognitive retraining assignment for depression:

Assignment	As applicable to a man who had been fired
1. Describing an upsetting situation.	Going on a job interview.
2. Identifying the emotions you feel.	Resentful, angry, anxious.
3. Listing your automatic thoughts.	I'll never find another job. It's hopeless. I got fired and nobody wants me.

| 4. Listing rational alternative responses | I've just started looking. I lost my job because of a merger. The culture and I didn't fit. It has nothing to do with my real abilities. People get hired for jobs every day of the year; it's only a matter of time until I get a new one too. |

(Source: R. C. Bedrosian and A. T. Beck, "Principles of Cognitive Therapy." In *Psychotherapy Process: Current Issues and Future Directions*. M. J. Mahoney, ed. New York: Plenum Press, 1980. As reprinted in *Abnormal Psychology: Current Perspectives*. R. R. Bootzin and T. R. Acocella. New York: Random House, 1988.)

Cognitive therapy may actually work even better than drug therapy for depression in some patients, both right after the treatment is over and on a long-term basis.

YOU ARE GETTING SLEEPY—OR HYPNOSIS

The room is dark, save for one spot of light illuminating the pocketwatch in the bearded therapist's hand. In a low monotone, he tells you to stare at the watch as it swings back and forth, back and forth. He tells you that you are getting sleepy . . . more and more sleepy. You go into a trance, powerless under the hypnotist's commands.

This scenario can be seen in almost every grade B horror movie since the genre first made it to the screen. The hypnotist is usually sinister; the victim is usually a young, pretty girl.

Unfortunately these myths have continued even today. Many of us have trepidation at the thought of going to a hypnotist. We are afraid of what we will do in our hypnotic state. We are afraid of relinquishing control.

But the real facts about hypnosis are vastly different from its Bela Lugosi image:

◢ We control the hypnosis; we determine whether we will "go under" from the hypnotist's power of suggestion.

⚡ We can come out of a hypnotic state any time we want.

⚡ Hypnosis is done by licensed, fully trained therapists who use it as any other therapautic tool to make you well.

⚡ Hypnosis is less of a trance-like state than it is a deep form of relaxation.

Hypnosis today has had success in treating bad habits that have resisted other therapy methods including overeating and smoking. As you go into a relaxed state, you become more susceptible to messages. A hypnotist will repeat various phrases to reinforce positive behavior: "Smoking is a terrible habit. . . . You really don't want to smoke. . . . You hate the smell. . . ."

Hypnosis is also used as a tool to create better self-images in anxious or depressed people. Here, the reinforcing messages might be "You have a great many good qualities"; "You like yourself"; "Whenever you have a negative thought about yourself, you will stop it in midstream"; "You are calm and worthy."

Self-hypnosis is becoming an increasingly popular tool for relaxation. "New-age" tapes that use relaxation techniques in combination with visualizations are part of many corporations' stress-management programs. All you do is plug in your Walkman, lie down and close your eyes. The tapes instruct you to relax your muscles, to release your tension, to picture anything from a balmy day on a sailboat to a deserted sandy beach. After approximately fifteen minutes, you are instructed to slowly open your eyes and "come back." More times than not, you are able to go about your business considerably less stressed.

Relaxation is important for aftershock victims too; the continuous "tapes" that replay the trauma create anxiety and panic that can build up to unmanageable proportions. By learning how to relax your muscles and your mind, you can help control these tapes—instead of their controlling you.

Hypnosis can also help re-create the trauma for people suffering from aftershock. What the conscious mind refuses to discuss can come up without inhibitions during a deeply relaxed state. And by reexperiencing the overwhelming pain and fear, an aftershock victim comes closer to abreaction, that crucial element of psychotherapy that helps put the trauma back into its rightful time and place, that helps one integrate the trauma into a new world view and get on with life.

> Here's a deep-breathing exercise to help you relax. Try it either lying down or sitting.
>
> **1**   Take several deep breaths, breathing in through your nose and out your mouth. Close your eyes.
>
> **2**   Imagine yourself on a deserted beach. The waves are soothing. The sun is bright and warm on your body.
>
> **3**   Take several more deep breaths as you picture this peaceful scene.
>
> **4**   You are now going to clench and unclench various parts of your body, clenching as you breathe in, releasing as you breathe out. Start with your eyes, squeezing them shut, move to your jaw, your neck, your shoulders . . . Continue moving down your body and finish with your toes.
>
> **5**   Take several more long deep breaths. Tense your entire body at once—then release. Do this one more time.
>
> **6**   Open your eyes. You should feel much more relaxed!

One final note: If you can't be hypnotized or if the trauma is so severely repressed that even hypnosis can't get it to surface, there is a therapy called narconanalysis that can help. Here, a psychiatrist will use sodium pentothol to re-create the traumatic event. Eventually, with repeated treatment, you will be able to desensitize the trauma and abreaction will naturally occur.

DO YOU WANT TO TALK ABOUT IT—OR GROUP THERAPY

"Why do you always come in here looking so defensive?"

"But you always seem so self-assured to me."

"That's exactly what happened to me."

"Sometimes I needed someone to understand so much, I thought I was going to go crazy."

"You really do know how I feel."

That's members of a group therapy session talking—many saying things they would never say outside their therapist's office. Learning to express your feelings to others is only one reason why group therapy is effective. The following points are derived from Irwin Yalom's book,

The Theory and Practice of Group Psychotherapy, second edition (Basic Books, 1975) as reprinted in *Abnormal Psychology: Current Perspectives*, fifth edition (Random House, 1988):

✓ *Education.* A member of the group can learn how to cope in the world after a rape, after a debilitating illness, after losing a loved one. He or she can learn strategies about handling pressure on the job, about assertiveness, about dealing with family and friends.

✓ *Hope.* Through the close connection of others in the same or in different struggles, a group member finds inspiration and hope that things can change.

✓ *Universality.* Through the experiences of others, a group member realizes that he or she is not fighting a battle alone.

✓ *Altruism.* By offering advice, sympathy, and encouragement to others, a group member understands first-hand that he or she has something to give—something valuable.

✓ *Family feelings.* A group supervised by a therapist is like a family with the parent at the helm; it offers the chance to heal old wounds and gain insight into a member's original family ties.

✓ *Social skills.* Honest feedback from others helps a group member develop interpersonal skills.

✓ *Role modeling.* Imitation is the highest form of flattery, and here in a group, a member can find an inspiring model (the group leader or another member) to change old, destructive behavior.

✓ *Experimenting.* A group can help members examine their values, seeing exactly what they want from a relationship, a job, and life itself. The comfortable setting offers a chance to try out "new selves" and new ways of behavior without fear.

✓ *Cohesiveness.* A group offers a sense of belonging and safety —an essential atmosphere for growth.

✓ *Catharsis.* Here in the comfort of the group, members can let loose about their feelings and their traumatic experiences. By expressing their bottled up emotions, members begin the journey toward putting the trauma back into its rightful time and place.

A crisis-intervention therapist will use group therapy to reinforce the insights an aftershock victim gains in individual therapy. A patient of mine was suffering from aftershock after his colostomy. He dealt with his feelings in therapy, but he learned how to exist in the world by joining a colostomy self-help group. A Vietnam vet suffering from the throes of war might be learning about his new realities in therapy, but he will get his understanding and empathy from a group of Vietnam vets. An executive suffering from the stress and strain of his highly visible, highly responsible job learns relaxation techniques and coping skills in his individual therapy. But he learns specific strategies about management from a self-help group that includes top executives from different fields. (Note: Executive groups usually consist of members from different professions, so as not to foster inhibitions or mistrust of competition. The group the executive in question joined included a professor, a doctor, a lawyer, and a fashion designer, none of whom would ever participate in his social sphere.)

Finally, group therapy can help a violent aftershock victim control his or her emotions. The likelihood of outbursts diminishes in a group setting, even as growth and understanding increase.

YOU SAY POTATO, I SAY POTATO—OR FAMILY AND COUPLES THERAPY

Aftershock is a family problem. Whether it's an alcoholic father, a depressed mother, or a hostile teenager, no one is excluded from the slings and arrows of traumatic pain. While working at the Connecticut Mental Health Center, Margaret Raymond (a social worker) and I identified seven stages of response that most families go through when a member is suffering from mental pain:

1. Uneasiness
2. Seeking reassurance
3. Denial and minimizing
4. Making the sick one an outsider
5. Feelings of guilt, shame, and grief
6. Confusion in the changed family situation
7. Acceptance of reality and the search for help

As these seven stages show, families suffer their own brand of aftershock when one of them gets sick. And the fastest way to move from stage one to stage seven is through family therapy. Here under the guidance of a therapist, family members can learn the facts about their sick member and how they can better understand and help. A study of eighteen recently released schizophrenics showed that if the family understood and supported their sick members, incidence of relapses was drastically curtailed. The eighteen families participated in family therapy, learning new ways to cope and to express their emotions, finding new strategies for handling crises that might come up, and understanding how important it was that the discharged patient take his or her medicine. After nine months, only one out of the eighteen schizophrenics was readmitted, as opposed to eight out of eighteen in a group that did not have family therapy.

In couples therapy, the key is in communication. If a husband, for example, is suffering from depression, the resentment, guilt, and shame the wife might feel as a result of that depression could seriously undermine the marriage, unless those feelings are expressed. A therapist can help her open up in front of her husband. He in turn can talk about his pain in front of his wife. The result is instant feedback and invaluable insights into each other's needs, values, and hopes. As a prominent couples therapist once said, "Most partners in a marriage communicate very little of what they are really thinking or feeling. Many times they aren't even sure themselves. The therapy format can give them the skills to, first, analyze what they are really feeling and what they really want, then, secondly, express those needs and feelings to each other."

SMILE, YOU'RE ON VIDEOTHERAPY

This therapy tool is exactly what its name implies, videotaping your sessions throughout the different stages of treatment. For many of us memory is selective; we only remember what we chose to remember. Let's say that three weeks into your therapy, you decide it isn't working, that you are not making progress and you are not feeling better at all. Looking at a videotape of your first session would change all that. There, in living color, is your pain and anxiety as it was; the way you feel, the way you look today is proof that you have indeed made progress.

Videotherapy is particularly effective in drug and alcohol rehabilitation. It can provide a "reality check" once your treatment is over.

Whether three months, four months, or one year later, if you reach a point where you say, "Well, it wasn't so bad; the drugs really didn't do me in" you only have to turn on your VCR and play your videocassette to realize you *were* that bad, that you are much better off today.

A fairly new technique, videotherapy has vast implications for the future as a reinforcement for positive behavior, as a teaching device, and as a reminder to the patient that he or she has had the courage and the stamina to get well—and stay well.

THE IRRATIONAL FEAR—OR ELECTROSHOCK THERAPY

Electroshock therapy has had a bad reputation for too long. Yes, it is a serious therapy. No, it is not used until other alternatives have been explored. Yes, it is used for severely depressed. But—

> ✏ Its positive results are seen immediately. Drug therapy takes anywhere from two to four weeks or longer to take effect. If time is a luxury a severely depressed person cannot afford, electro-shock can be the answer.
>
> ✏ The ability to learn new material comes back almost imme-diately. Within a few weeks, all memory is intact.
>
> ✏ The depressed patient is given anesthesia before the shock therapy; it does not hurt.
>
> ✏ Today's innovations in medicine and science assure success. In many cities, electroshock treatment can even be given on an outpatient basis.

These then are some of the techniques available in the 1980s to treat the disease of aftershock. All of them, at one time or another, have been used in various combinations in crisis-intervention therapy. To give you an idea of how they work, let us observe a crisis-interven-tion therapy program in action.

THE SCENE

Ellen had lost her husband suddenly four years ago. She was thirty-two at the time of his death. At first she seemed to handle the loss well; she went through an initial grieving period of several months, then gradually went back to her routines. At first, when she began to cry for no apparent reason, she assumed it was nothing; she was still mourning. But then her crying bouts became more severe. One time she began crying on the bus going home from work. She cried at her desk. And in the evenings she cried almost continuously. Ellen began to act compulsively. She placed her husband's picture by her bed and talked to it. She refused to get rid of his clothes. She began to have terrible nightmares. Her husband would appear, smiling, his arms opened wide; suddenly his expression would change. He would try to kill her.

Things went from bad to worse. Ellen couldn't go out with any other men. She had no interest in sex. Her appetite decreased and she lost weight. She kept calling in sick at work. She began to make dinners for herself and her husband, setting his place at the table. She began to spend more and more time alone. Ellen's aftershock symptoms were consuming her. She could no longer function in her daily life. After two years of pain, a woman friend insisted she get help.

THE TREATMENT

Here, step-by-step, is the therapeutic process Ellen experienced, based on the treatment outlined in Dr. C. B. Scrignar's book, *Posttraumatic Stress Disorder* (Praeger, 1984).

1. *Individual psychotherapy.* **At the outset—and during her entire therapeutic process—Ellen met with her therapist to discuss, to learn, and to grow. The first order of business: ventilation. In the first few visits, it was crucial she discuss her husband's death to relive the pain she felt when she first got the news.**

2. *Hypnosis and relaxation exercises.* **Ellen had a hard time ventilating. Consequently, her therapist taught her how to use hypnosis and deep relaxation to open up and find the ability to express her emotions.**

3. *Differential diagnosis.* **After careful testing Ellen's therapist determined she was suffering from aftershock.**

4. *Education.* **Ellen's therapist carefully explained that she was suffering from aftershock and why. He explained that she never went through the necessary stages of grief and acceptance, that she continued to play her trauma in her head.**

5   *Drug therapy.* Ellen was given Xanax to relieve her anxiety about leaving the house. She was given a tricyclic called imipramine to ease her depression. She was carefully monitored throughout her therapy.

6   *Behavioral modification therapy.* Ellen was taught to change the negative "videotapes" in her head using thought-changing techniques, imagery, and four positive reinforcing statements:

    ⚡ I feel uncomfortable.
    ⚡ I have had these feelings before and nothing ever happened.
    ⚡ There is nothing seriously wrong with me.
    ⚡ I am experiencing anxiety and will practice my relaxation techniques.

7   *Abreaction.* In her individual therapy, Ellen reached the point where she was able to relive her husband's death and accept it.

8   *Systematic desensitizing.* Ellen's fear of death was put to rest through seeing various images of death in her therapist's office while she was in a relaxed state.

9   *Family therapy.* Ellen's parents and sister were brought in for counseling and education, to learn how they could best support her.

10   *Group therapy.* Ellen joined a group of young widows and learned she was not alone.

11   *Assertiveness training.* In a group environment, Ellen learned how to gain control of her life with assertiveness, not aggression.

12   *Problem solving.* Within her individual sessions, Ellen discussed the various problems that came up in her other therapies: her relationship with the others in her group, her resentments and love for her family, her ability to act assertively, and her hopes and fears for the future.

13   *Exercise and nutrition.* Ellen was put on a health routine to further calm her emotions, improve her outlook, and ease the stress of her everyday life.

14   *Self-assessment.* In her individual therapy, Ellen realized that the world was not all black or white; she realized that she was not in pain all the time, that she was a survivor, not a victim of fate.

15   *Work*. Ellen was recovering at a good pace. She went back to work and slowly began re-entering her world.

16   *Socializing*. Ellen was asked out one night by an attractive man she met on the commuter train. She said yes.

Today one year later, Ellen is engaged to be married. She is off her medication; she has received a promotion at work. She is no longer in therapy, but she has joined a health club and is a member of a support group for executive women.

IS THE CURE WORTH THE PAIN?

Does therapy work? There are those who believe that psychiatric conditions can be cured by time. But in a study done at Temple University's outpatient clinic, 80 percent of the patients who went for therapy improved—as opposed to only 48 percent among those who were not treated.

Yes, storms can be weathered. Times do change. But aftershock can get worse if left untreated. If therapy can bring you hope for the future, time to live up to your potential, and freedom from your anxious days and nights, the answer to the above question has to be a resounding yes.

You have now learned exactly what aftershock is and why it occurs. You have discovered some of the pressure points in today's world that can cause its pain. You have seen the different therapies at work that can stop it in its tracks.

But it is not yet time to say good-bye. The most important element of aftershock is yet to come: prevention. You can live freely and happily in an aftershock world. You can find the means to keep its stress at bay. And in the next section I will show you how to do just that.

PART FOUR:

LIVING WELL AND HAPPY IN A SHOCKING WORLD

AN OUNCE OF PREVENTION

> *Stress is as necessary to see the structure of the personality*
> *as tension is to see the structure of a crystal.*
> —SIGMUND FREUD

A WOMAN WHO SURVIVED A TERRIBLE PLANE CRASH talked to me and Dr. Glicksman about her experiences. Listen to the following dialogue:

> QUESTION: Did it change your values at all? Have you found that you appreciate life more in any way or less in any way than you did?
>
> PATIENT: Oh [yes], I was always very family oriented, to my own kids particularly. . . . They have been very, very important to me. I think that probably one reason I got better was I had to get home to take care of the kids.
>
> QUESTION: You really felt that the need to be . . . that you were wanted and needed played a role?
>
> PATIENT: The one thing that I always felt I was good at and I really loved [was] being a mother, so I'm sure that was very primary in my mind . . . to hurry up and get home so things could

get back to normal. People are much more important to me than they were before, and I can't say it's a drastic change for me because I've always appreciated nature and people . . . but I think it's greater, much greater.

A reason to live—the ultimate motivation to get well and to stay well. We have discussed the therapist's role in helping you find a raison de vivre for life. We have talked about the importance of friends or family to help you through the worst of a crisis. And we have learned to see a crisis as a window of opportunity, a chance to grow and gain important insights about yourself, about your loved ones, and about life itself. George Eliot once wrote that "The strongest principle in growth lies in human potential." Like the patient above, we all have that potential inside us—to grow, to be the very best we can be, and to come through a crisis intact.

Reducing the stress in your life is one way of coping with a turbulent world. The stress you feel right now has a direct correlation to the way you will handle a crisis—and whether or not you develop aftershock. Our opportunities for growth are out there. With understanding, you can grab hold of them and flourish.

Take a moment to check off the list below. It will help you determine whether you are feeling the debilitating effects of stress and to see the areas in your life that need improvement.

THE SIGNS OF STRESS

Check every item that pertains to you. Be honest. There are no right or wrong answers, only behavioral symptoms of stress that can be changed for good.

☐ 1   Drink more than three cups of coffee a day.
☐ 2   Always seem to skip meals.
☐ 3   Don't bother taking vitamins.
☐ 4   End up doing everything myself.
☐ 5   Blow up at the slightest provocation.
☐ 6   Never seem to reach my goals.
☐ 7   Have no long-term plans for the future.

8 Haven't had a good laugh in a long time.

9 Ignore my body's aches and pains.

10 Blow everything out of proportion.

11 See things as black and white—with no shades of gray.

12 Never seem to relax.

13 Am completely disorganized.

14 Avoid new people and situations.

15 Never show my emotions.

16 Hate to exercise.

17 Don't have any friends I can really trust.

18 Feel out of control.

19 Have every minute and every hour designated in my planner.

20 Can't sleep.

21 Can't get up in the morning.

22 Never had a massage.

23 Start to get angry when someone is even five minutes late.

24 Keep putting things off.

25 Think about the good old days a lot.

26 Have no spiritual outlet.

27 Haven't had a physical checkup in years.

28 Smoke too much.

29 Drink too much.

30 Find getting dressed up and groomed a chore.

31 Have one way—the right way—to do things.

32 Never let myself go.

33 Think everyone is expendable.

34 Say yes to everything.

35 Race through my days.

36 Gossip.

37 Hate any kind of routine.

38 Always seem to be in the middle of a crisis.

39 Ignore the way my home and office looks.

40 Sit back and let things happen.

41 Never take vacations.

42 Discount the new technology, from computers to compact discs.

43 Get so upset about things during the day that I stay up thinking about them all night long.

44 Overeat to ease my anxiety.

45 Feel nauseated and have diarrhea often.

46 Have people in my life that make me feel uptight.

Add up all your checkmarks. The closer you are to forty-six, the more stress you are experiencing in your life and the more you need to develop better coping skills.

THE THREE Cs

Why do some people handle stress better than others? In her study of American executives across the country published in *American Health*, Dr. Suzanne Ouellette Kobasa found three character traits that help reduce the stress of traumatic shock:

⚡ *Commitment* to yourself, your work, your values, and your family

⚡ *Control* over your own life

⚡ *Challenging* life's crises as situations to master

The patient who talked about her family in the beginning of the chapter instinctively understood these three Cs. She came through her trauma successfully. But there are ways to develop these character strengths, even if you are currently in the midst of a traumatic event and feeling out of control.

Take up something you can control. The smallest task, when it has been accomplished, will immediately make you feel better and more in control. If you are feeling overwhelmed, try taking up some physical exercise. Finish walking that mile. Do those errands you have been putting off: that baby present, the dry cleaners, that obligatory phone call. Change your focus. If your stress is from the office, focus on your life at home. If your stress is at home, focus on your work.

Find a challenge you can master. If your stressful life event is so over-whelming that even to contemplate it is too much, find something you *can* master. Learn how to use a computer. Take tennis lessons. Learn a foreign language. Mastering these challenges will not only make you feel better but can give you the confidence to challenge and master your crisis.

Take some time to analyze the stressful event. Think about the precipitating event. How could you have handled it better? And more important, how could you have handled it worse? Putting things in their proper perspective helps you get a grip on them. It helps emphasize the positive and show you new ways to cope.

Try to keep a routine. Knowing that you are doing things according to plan helps control your panic. If you are keeping the same hours every day, if you are organized, and if you allow time for rest, you can gain the comfort of knowing that some aspects of your life are normal, that despite your crisis life is moving on. To help keep that routine going, try to eat right and exercise. These disciplines will reduce routine-destroying tension.

Share your fears and doubts with others. Don't underestimate the value of support. Sympathy and understanding go a long way toward helping you push through a crisis. By talking over your problems, you can circumvent misunderstanding. You can release some of those bottled up emotions. You can find needed comfort. If family or friends are too far away to help on a continuous basis, join a support group. There is even greater comfort in numbers.

Seek help. The earlier your therapy starts, the faster and better it will work. Period.

STOPPING STRESS

It's a fact we have gone over again and again; traumatic events are a part of life. We can't control them, but we can learn how to handle them better. The preceding pages were designed to help you do just that. Now, join me in learning how to deal with a trauma *before* it strikes. Together we can

⚡ Cope with shocking events when they occur,
⚡ Stop aftershock in its tracks,
⚡ Enjoy the positive traumas to their fullest,
⚡ Reduce the pain of negative traumas, and
⚡ Build up strength and resilience—and grow.

It's called prevention and it's not magic. It's all about making the stress of daily life work for you. In the next chapter, I will be going over my step-by-step strategies for living in a shocking, stress-filled world. They have worked for me, my patients, and countless others. They can work for you. And that's the shocking truth.

STOPPING STRESS STEP-BY-STEP

Considering how dangerous everything is,
nothing is really very frightening!
—GERTRUDE STEIN

THINK ABOUT IT: IF WE DIDN'T HAVE THE STRESS to pay our bills, we would never be motivated to work, and we would lose the opportunity to achieve. If we didn't have the stress of deadlines, we would never finish anything, and we would never know the satisfaction of a job well done. If we didn't have the stress of staying healthy, we would never quit bad habits, and we would find our lives cut in half. If we didn't have the stress of our need to love, we would never have an intimate relationship, and we would never discover the pleasures of romance. If we didn't have the stress of daily life, we would never take risks, and we would never discover who we are or what we want.

Stress is not bad. It is not the evil by-product of the 1980s. *It is how we handle that stress that makes it bad.* Stress can be the thing that pushes us over the edge or the springboard to growth and opportunity. At some point it will be up to us to choose the path either of destruction or of self-fulfillment.

STRATEGIES FOR STRESS MANAGEMENT

To live is to feel stress, whether it comes from the pressure points of your job, your personal life, or the world at large. It's up to you to make stress work against you—or for you. The following strategies were designed to make stress an ally. They offer alternatives to that downward spiral called aftershock. They can help you cope in a stress-filled world and prevent future shock for good. As a wise sage once said, "Better to aim for the sky and hit a star, than aim for the fence and hit the dirt." Aim high. Here's how.

1. Choosing friends who will support and encourage you. We have already discussed how friends can give you needed support and encouragement during a stressful crisis. But they can also help you cope with day-to-day stress.

Picture the following scenario. You have had a hard day at work and you have a splitting migraine. If you go home, you will pull the covers over your head and feel the pain the long night through. But if you meet a friend after work, there is less time to think about your migraine. You get distracted, and your headache goes away. Friends can soften both the major and the minor blows of life.

But good friends can be hard to find. We have talked about how friends help shape your psychological identity, how they can inspire confidence and self-esteem or feelings of rejection. Only friends who share your values and understand your needs can help you cope with stress. Look over the values quiz in Chapter Ten. Think about your answers. If you discover you love to cook, why not take a course in gourmet lo-cal dining? If you are fascinated by horseback riding, why not try a dude ranch weekend? People whose values match yours are out there. They, too, need close friends.

2. Not putting off till tomorrow what you can do today. In her book, *Feel the Fear and Do It Anyway* (Harcourt Brace Jovanovich, 1987) Dr. Susan Jeffers says that "Pushing through fear is less frightening than living with the underlying fear that comes from a feeling of helplessness." If you keep postponing the study time you need to pass an exam, the pressure and anxiety about failing will just keep building. Soon you won't have the time to study at all and you could find yourself with a self-fulfilling prophecy on your hands. Do it now. Relieve your stress and get it done. Remember the people I talked about in connection with cognitive therapy in Chapter Twelve? They found that their anxiety about a task never matched the reality of the situation—which always expended much less energy than they had thought.

3. *Leaving the past behind.* We all have pasts—some filled with fond memories and some so upsetting we still dwell on them today. But good, bad, or ugly, the past is still the past. We can't bring someone back to life, and we can't undo mistakes. Why create stress over something we cannot change? View the past as a teacher. Learn from past mistakes. Focus on what could have done better and what could have done worse. (See Chapter Thirteen.) Look ahead instead of back. Your future can still be changed.

4. *Getting physical.* If you don't address the stress in your life, it won't go away. If you try to ignore your anxiety and your fatigue, they won't stay under wraps. Instead, your stress will manifest itself in physical illness, from headaches and high blood pressure to depression and hives. If you continue to miss meals because you are always on the go, you can develop hypoglycemia, a low blood sugar condition that can make you irritable and anxious. If you grab sweet, sugary snacks to keep you going, you can find yourself with sugar blues, complete with dangerous mood swings. If you stay up all night because your mind is going around and around, you may be not only a victim of insomnia but also susceptible to flus and colds.

But you can cancel your date with aftershock by getting enough exercise and sleep, by taking vitamins and eating nutritionally, and by avoiding too much caffeine and alcohol. One good habit begets another. As you begin to exercise, your body releases endorphins—natural tranquilizers that will help you sleep. And after a good night's sleep you will wake up refreshed and more in control. That good feeling, in turn, will keep you going, so you won't have to grab a sweet to stay awake. Soon, before you know it, your moods will even out.

The Greeks found moderation the key to a good life. But moderation does not mean abstinence. There is no reason why you can't have that chocolate-rich dessert when you are out to dinner. There is no reason why you can't celebrate your promotion with champagne. But to cope better with the stress of everyday life, combine your pleasure with a regular exercise routine and low-fat, low-sugar foods. You will not only better appreciate the celebrations of life, but you will have more energy and more zest for your everyday routines.

5. *Avoiding impossible dreams.* We all need goals to think about, to keep us going, and to give us a reason to live. We need to dream to experience life. But trying to fulfill unrealistic goals will only be an added stress. Saying you will hand in the proposal by the end of the week when you really need two weeks is only going to set you up for failure and its inherent stress. Dreaming of a chateau in the south of France when you can barely make the rent on your apartment will only make you depressed and stop you from getting out of a bad situation. Remember the Alcoholics Anonymous serenity prayer that I mentioned earlier? To repeat: "Lord, grant me the courage to change what I can, the serenity to accept what I cannot, and the wisdom to know the difference." Options are not unlimited. Make goals that reflect your lifestyle, your age, and your circumstances.

6. *Knowing your values.* When Shakespeare wrote "To thine own-self be true," he knew what he was talking about. If you don't understand what your strengths, weaknesses, and values are, you will run into problems not only with your family and friends, but with yourself. A patient of mine named Helen desperately wanted to meet someone and marry. Though she was a country girl at heart, she lived in New York City, where she felt the statistics were in her favor. She came to me because she was unhappy and feeling the stress of city life. I helped her see that she could only change what she herself controlled. She couldn't make someone love her, but she could find a better, stress-free life for herself outside the city. Finally Helen moved to the suburbs, and within a few months she met a man, fell in love, and got happily married. The moral? Stay true to what your values are—and you will find that things work out.

Take time out to make lists of what you want and where you want to be a year and five years from now. Think what others have complimented you on in the past. Do you handle pressure well? Are you friendly? Think of the criticisms you have received. Do you procrastinate? Do you fly off the handle? Concentrate on your strengths. You are not all bad. Analyze your weaknesses; they can be changed. Remember Helen; being true to yourself will not only help you gain control over your life and reduce your everyday stress—but may just help you find that elusive thing called happiness as well.

7. *Not saying yes when you mean no.* No one enjoys feeling like a victim. But if you continuously say yes to everyone and everything, you will end up a self-sacrificing and stress-filled victim. Think about it. The last time you took on extra work, didn't you feel some resentment halfway through? Didn't you feel angry and depressed when you were forced to go to that party you had no desire to attend? Many times, our unconscious desires to be liked and avoid confrontations make us say yes when we really mean no. But, in the long run, this obligeance doesn't make people like us more, and because we have let our resentments simmer, more times than not they boil over into unpleasant confrontations. Try saying no—nicely. Don't give an answer right away. Instead, take some time to think about it. Write down your reply. Rehearse your response beforehand. You will find it easier to say no than you thought. And as an added plus, you will discover that your no is indeed respected.

8. *Getting angry!* "I'm mad as hell and I'm not going to take it anymore!" That was Peter Finch talking in his famous *Network* scene. It worked for him and it can work for you. I'm not recommending that you get angry at the slightest provocation (that, in itself, is a sign of stress); but expressing your feelings in an appropriate manner is a crucial stress reducer. Ventilation in therapy is one of the first steps toward health. It works the same way in everyday life. By letting out the steam, you can keep anxiety and tension at bay.

9. *Talking things over with supportive people.* The Japanese have many of the same bad habits that we do: They work too hard, they smoke, they drink, they have high blood pressure, they work under stress-filled conditions—and yet they live much longer than us. Why? Studies suggest that it's because they have close ties with their families, their friends, and their communities.

We have already discussed the importance of support groups. Informally or in a therapeutic environment, a group of people bound by similar experiences can offer insight and encouragement. Bounce your ideas off them. Talk about your problems. They can help you cope with the daily stresses in your life.

Today, there are thousands of support groups dealing with 270 conditions from alcoholism to weight disorders. In fact, one source found that 15 million Americans are members of one support group or another. Check your phone book or call your local community center or hospital to find a group to suit your needs. The legwork will be well worth the rewards.

10. Visualizing. Picture this in your mind's eye: You are in your usual meeting, talking as customary about your projections for next month. But this time, you are not looking down at the notes the whole time you speak. Your voice isn't mumbly, and you make eye contact with everyone in the room. Or picture this: You are in your favorite Mexican restaurant, enjoying the company of a friend you often go there with. But this time, you don't order the second fattening margarita and eat all the Nacho chips. You are in control of what you eat and drink, and you don't worry about going off yet another diet again.

These images are not far-fetched fantasies. They are examples of constructive visualization, a method of changing your behavior and making stressful situations work for you. Focusing on ways to cope with potential trouble zones can help you deal with them when they occur. If you can't imagine yourself acting any other way but anxiously, think of the ways someone you admire would handle it. Learning how to respond to stressful cues before they occur is just as important as . . .

11. Avoiding potentially stressful situations. If rush-hour traffic makes you want to scream, it makes perfect sense to leave work an hour later. If there is a nonessential meeting you dread going to, it's smart to send a coworker in your place. If you hate standing in line for anything, there is no reason why you shouldn't schedule that movie or those necessary errands for less crowded times of day. If the anticipation of early-morning appointments gives you insomnia and indigestion the night before, it's only sensible to make your important appointments for the afternoon. Avoiding stressful situations when you can doesn't mean you are running away from your problems. But it can make all the difference between a stress-filled day and a peaceful one.

12. Laughing. In his book, *Anatomy of an Illness* (W. W. Norton, 1979), Norman Cousins wrote about the role humor played in his miraculous recovery from a terminal spinal disease. Hospitals across the country have set up humor programs to help their patients deal with their crippling illnesses.

Laughter is indeed the best medicine. If we can find humor in the things we can't control in our day-to-day struggles to survive, we can indeed conquer the heavy weight of stress. As Oscar Wilde once said, "Life is far too important to take seriously."

13. Being polite. A simple thank you, a soft excuse me, a courteous smile, an opened door. Actions can speak louder than words. An act of kind politeness can go a long way to making you feel better about yourself. And if you are polite in turn, your self-image will continue to be enhanced.

14. Being well groomed. Billy Crystal might get well-deserved laughs when he says, "You look good, you feel good." But in humor there is truth. The fact is that dressing well commands respect. It's a sign of confidence and a sign of self-control—two silent affirmations that you are on your way to reducing stress.

15. Learning to be flexible. The best-laid plans can often go awry. You can plan and plan for a vacation—but you can't foresee the kids coming down with chicken pox. You can spend two days and two nights slaving over a report on an innovative product—only to find that your boss has decided to put all new business on hold. You can organize your day to the best of your ability—only to get called in for an emergency meeting that just can't wait.

Life is full of obstacles. The iron fist approach that promotes rigid thinking also promotes additional stress. There are other ways to do things. You are not always right. Very few things in life turn out the way we plan. A little flexibility can make all the difference between spending your time feeling miserable, or spending it constructively by putting other options to work.

16. Being assertive. Your family, friends, and colleagues make up your world. They can bring great joy into your life—or great stress when things are less than harmonious. Occasional tension between friends and loved ones is normal; it is a part of the dynamics of interpersonal relationships. But that friction can add undue stress if ignored. Communicating how you feel is important. Getting your opinions and your needs across in an effective, nonforceful way is called assertiveness. It means taking the time to think about what you want to say. It means venting your anger constructively—and calmly. Aggression will only turn people off and create even more stress than you already have. But explaining things in an assertive manner will not only clear the air, it will reduce your tense feelings considerably. Don't be a passive victim. Don't look to others to change their ways. Take charge! All you have to lose is your stress.

17. Delegating responsibility. There has been a shift in the marketplace. It used to be that the employees who stayed late were the ones slated for promotion. Today the practice is considered a sign of poor management. If you must stay till all hours to complete your work, it means you don't know how to manage people very well. Smart people delegate work to others on the job—and at home. The tasks get done in half the time, leaving you stress-free. The rewards? More time for long-range planning at work and more time for pleasure at home.

18. Relaxing. We have already discussed the fight-or-flight response that leads to aftershock. That same chemical imbalance can create a continuous state of stress, leading to high blood pressure, tension headaches, muscle cramps, and tremors.

But you can stop the debilitating effects of stress—with regular, programmed relaxation. Doing muscle relaxation exercises as discussed in Chapter Twelve can recirculate your blood back to your extremities, and away from fight-or-flight stressed muscles. Taking a few moments a day to relax your mind with a relaxation or self-hypnosis tape will quiet your brain's fight-or-flight cassette. Studies have proved that meditation can relieve stress and increase productivity; metabolism, blood pressure, and heart rate all slow down.

Other relaxation techniques include massage, yoga, and biofeedback. All give you a break from your hectic schedule; all put you in touch with your anatomy and your emotions; all offer you time out to revitalize, recharge, and reacquaint yourself with body and soul.

One important tip: Start your relaxation schedule when you are calm. If you aren't feeling stressed, it will work much more successfully the first few times out. Success then breeds success; when you really need your relaxation method to calm you down, it will!

19. Slowing down. "Slow down, you're movin' too fast. Gotta make the moment last . . ." was the mainstay of a generation twenty years ago. Simon and Garfunkel were "Feelin' Groovy," but in the 1980s world, who has time? The fact is you *must* make time to slow down. If you don't, your body just might do it for you—with a heart attack, an accident, or a bad flu. It's well worth the effort to put on your answering machine, block off some hours in your calendar, shut the office door, or run off for a warm, relaxing weekend in the sun. In addition to reducing your stress, there is the added benefit of fun!

20. Concentrating on the small steps. There is an ancient Buddhist saying: "The journey of a thousand miles begins with one step." Sometimes dwelling on the total picture causes so much stress that you never make that first move. Sometimes you lose your determination and stamina along the way and never make it to your journey's end. One way to avoid these scenarios is to formulate subgoals that in the long run add up to what you want accomplished. Margaret, for example, wanted to lose forty pounds. But the thought of losing all that weight sabotaged her time and again. Then she made her goal five pounds and was able to meet the challenge with no problem. Losing those five pounds motivated her to lose another five, and within six months she was down to her target weight.

Margaret is not alone. Let's say your goal is to become physically fit. If you quit smoking, begin a strict diet, and start an almost impossible exercise regime all at the same time, you will be setting yourself up for failure. The stress would be impossible to handle. But if you made quitting smoking your first priority, followed a month or so later with moderate exercise and a sensible diet, you will not only reach your goal—but you will get there with a lot less pain.

Alcoholics Anonymous says it best: "One day at a time." Those small first steps will eventually turn into that one big step that had been so terrifying.

21. Bringing spirituality into your life. It doesn't have to be God. It can be friendship or love. It can be the new-age searching for inner peace. But whatever it is, religion should not be underestimated. Belief in a higher power helps in the face of stress; it transcends your immediate pain. Not only does a sense of spirituality provide a link between the past, the present, and the future, it offers a continuum, a solid place in the family of man. As Dante wrote in *Paradiso,* "In His will is our tranquility." Amen.

22. Managing your time. Time can be a most precious gift—or a spy from an enemy camp. It all depends on how well you manage yours. You can't make more hours in the day, but you can adjust them to reduce stress and enjoy them more. Here are some hints:

✔ Set up only half the hours in your day to fit in those unexpected meetings or emergencies.

✔ Balance your day judiciously. Leave time for family and friends. Balance is the key to a less stressful life.

✔ Use a month-at-a-glance calendar. You can see immediately how your schedule is stacking up. If things get too crowded, stop scheduling for the month!

✔ Analyze the plans you make. Will you have enough time between appointments to regroup? Did you take traveling time into account? Think before you say yes.

23. *Organizing and setting priorities.* Not everything must be done today. Make daily lists of what you would like to accomplish that day. Put an asterisk by the tasks that must be done; the others can always be transferred to tomorrow's daily list. If you make your list the night before, you won't spend half the night worrying about what you have to do. It's all there in black and white on your night table.

To organize means to plan. Set up meetings that take place in the same part of town, so you don't spend half your day running back and forth. Try to do several errands at one time. If you get to the dry cleaners, the drugstore, and the shoemaker in the same hour block of time, you will feel as if you have expended less energy—and less stress —for those routine chores that, though necessary, can build up and weigh you down.

24. *Being spontaneous.* Children know the secret of a happy life; they are spontaneous. Unencumbered with responsibility, they can be free to explore, discover, and delight in joyful abandon. But even as adults, we can lose control for brief moments at a time. Listening to a masterful symphony; enjoying the pleasures of sex; walking through a gallery filled with great works of art; sitting back against a tree on a hot summer day. Let go. Relish your loss of control. It is these times that proclaim and reaffirm the celebration of life.

These are only some strategies for making stress work for you. Think about the ways you have coped in the past. They can help you formulate your own strategies, your own set of coping skills that, in combination with these twenty-four steps, can become your individual recipe for stress success.

Remember, the whole is much greater than its parts. When you make physical changes, they help promote changes in the way you think. When you change your work environment, those changes will follow through at home. When you change the ways you manage time, you can make changes in your personal relationships. One change begets another. Soon your whole world can be stress free.

Listen to your body and your soul. Take heart. As the saying goes, "Ships in harbor are safe, but that's not what ships are built for." Take sail today.

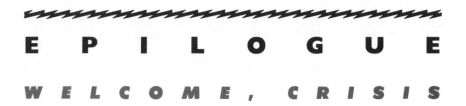

E P I L O G U E

W E L C O M E ,   C R I S I S

T HE CHINESE CHARACTER FOR CRISIS COMBINES both the figures for danger and opportunity. It is no accident then, that an ancient Chinese proverb states: "Welcome crises." But to Western eyes, it would seem strange to welcome what we consider dangerous. After all, none of us would welcome an unexpected death or an eroding marriage. None of us would welcome illness or a stock market crash. And as we have seen, even positive crises are not always greeted with welcoming arms and profuse tears of joy. A mother cries at the sight of her healthy newborn baby. Another woman dreads going to work the first day after her promotion. A man slinks into depression at the sight of his new home.

Yet all these crises can mean growth. A crisis by definition is a turning point in anything. It can turn us toward an optimistic future— or leave us feeling aftershock in the dust. Which will it be for us in the eighties?

That these are strange times is not in doubt—but then, the times have always been strange. In World War II, the British and the Germans played chess with each other on Christmas Eve, only to resume fighting the next day. The great plagues would never have reached epidemic proportions had it not been for the continuous raping and pillaging—all done in the name of God. Caesar created the greatest empire in the ancient world—and was stabbed for his trouble by the senators he made powerful. Moses led the Israelites through the desert for forty years to find their promised land—and was stopped from entering its border himself. Women wore poisonous lead-based makeup for centuries—even though they had seen proof that it caused disfigurement and early death.

And today? We have a world where, in their desire for American culture, the Japanese have flooded America with their nationals, only to bring them home because they are getting too Americanized. We have craved to see the glories of old world Europe, only to find them dotted with fast-food restaurants and suburbs that look like home. We are called the affluent society, but there are more homeless in America than ever before. We work harder and more energetically than we ever have, but we spend our nights dreaming of empty spaces and deserted islands. We go to the movies to escape, and watch postnuclear, war-action adventures. We want to escape, but we don't dare try. We want to be loved, but we are terrified to make that first move. We want a wonderful relationship, but we have impossible expectations.

Yes, life is fraught with irony. Yes, we live in a world where crises seem unrelenting. Yes, we do indeed live in turbulent times. But it is this very transient nature of our world that makes it *imperative* to make good choices with our lives.

And think of it: Today we also have more options than ever before. People can make a statement of who they want to be by choosing a psychological family that fulfills more of their needs than their own flesh and blood. People are choosing to reach out and deal with the world exactly as it is, turning away from racism, brutality, and the desire for war.

Yes, crises will always be among us. It then falls to us to let them lead us *away* from aftershock and welcome them for opportunities to grow.

Our journey here is almost at an end. We have learned together

216

the characteristics of our 1980s world. We have seen the elements that make up the traumas of our lives. We have discovered exactly what aftershock is—and who is more susceptible to its slings and arrows. We have seen the pressure points that bulk so large in our personal lives, our business lives, and our world at large. And together we have traveled back up from aftershock, through the advances in pharmaceutical medicines, and crisis-intervention therapies.

Together, we have seen the ways to avoid aftershock and the stress that always joins it. What is left?

Only this: a message for the future, for a world where we can live up to our full potential without fear, without anxiety, without the past to haunt our days.

Together, we can conquer the 1980s disease of aftershock. Together, we can make stress work for us. Together, we can welcome the world of crisis, a world of change—for the better.

For without these crises, there would be no life. And without life, there would be no hope.

Welcome, then, with me, crisis. We may never conquer death, but we can conquer life and make it the best it can be.

Together we can stop aftershock for good.

Welcome to a brave—and exciting—new world.

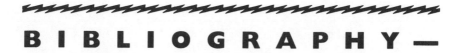

BIBLIOGRAPHY—

CHAPTER-BY-CHAPTER SOURCES

INTRODUCTION: AFTERSHOCK—GROWTH THROUGH CRISIS

Ettedgui, Eva, M.D. and Bridges, Mary, M.D. "Posttraumatic Stress Disorder," *Psychiatric Clinics of North America*, Vol. 8, No. 1, March 1985.

Jeffers, Susan, Ph.D. *Feel the Fear and Do It Anyway*, Harcourt Brace Jovanovich, 1987.

Slaby, Andrew E., M.D., Ph.D., and Glicksman, Arvin S., M.D. *Adapting to Life-Threatening Illness*, Praeger, 1985.

I. AFTERSHOCK—A SIGN OF THE TIMES

Canby, Vincent. "The Sorrows of Affluence" (Film Review of "Ordinary People,") *The New York Times*, September 19, 1980.

Mendelson, George. "The Concept of Posttraumatic Stress Disorder: A Review," *International Journal of Law and Psychiatry*, Vol. 10, 45–62, 1987.

2. WHAT IS TRAUMA?

American Psychiatric Association: *Diagnostic and Statistical Manual of Mental Disorders*, Third Edition, Revised, Washington, D.C., American Psychiatric Association, 1987.

Antilla, Susan. "Merger Traumatizes E. F. Hutton Workers," *USA Today*, December 21, 1987.

Raymond, Margaret Elmendorf, M.S.W.; Slaby, Andrew Edmund, M.D., M.P.H., and Lieb, Julian, M.D. *The Healing Alliance*, W. W. Norton & Company, Inc., 1975.

Winerip, Michael. "Where the Rich Find Comfort in Each Other," *The New York Times*, March 1, 1988.

3. WHAT IS AFTERSHOCK?

American Psychiatric Association: *Diagnostic and Statistical Manual of Mental Disorders*, Third Edition, Revised. Washington, D.C., American Psychiatric Association, 1987.

Brown, G., and Harris, T. *Social Origin of Depression: The Study of Psychiatric Disorders in Women*. London: Tavistock Publications, 1978.

Ettedgui, E., and Bridges, M. "Posttraumatic Stress Disorder," *Psychiatric Clinics of North America*, Vol. 8, No. 1, March 1985.

Garb, R., et al. "Varieties of Combat Stress Reaction: An Immunological Metaphor," *British Journal of Psychiatry*, No. 151, 248–51, 1987.

Horowitz, Mardi J., M.D. "Stress-Response Syndromes: A Review of Posttraumatic and Adjustment Disorders," *Hospital and Community Psychiatry*, Vol. 37, No. 3, March 1986.

Kelly, William E., M.D., editor. *Posttraumatic Stress Disorder and the War Veteran Patient*, Brunner/Mazel, Inc., 1985.

Kübler-Ross, Elisabeth, M.D. *On Death and Dying*, Macmillan, 1969.

Mendelson, George. "The Concept of Posttraumatic Stress Disorder: A Review," *International Journal of Law and Psychiatry*, Vol. 10, 45–62, 1987.

Pitman, Roger K. "Posttraumatic Stress Disorder, Conditioning, and Network Theory," *Psychiatric Annals*, Vol. 18, No. 3, March 1988.

Scrignar, C. B., M.D. *Posttraumatic Stress Disorder: Diagnosis, Treatment, and Legal Issues*, Praeger, 1984.

Van der Kolk, Bessel. A., M.D. "Trauma and Chronic Anxiety," *The Psychiatric Times*, 31–32, January 1988.

4. AFTERSHOCK SYMPTOMS

Dohrenwend, Barbara Snell and Dohrenwend, Bruce P. "Life Stress and Illness: Formulation of the Issues," *Stressful Life Events and Their Contexts* edited by Barbara Snell Dohrenwend and Bruce P. Dohrenwend, Prodist, 1981.

Fairbank, John A. and Nicholson, Robert A. "Theoretical and Empirical Issues in the Treatment of Posttraumatic Stress Disorder in Vietnam Veterans," *Journal of Clinical Psychology*, Vol. 43, No. 1, January 1987.

Gold, Mark S., M.D. *The Good News About Depression: Cures and Treatments in the New Age of Psychiatry*, Villard Books, 1987.

Mechanic, David, Ph.D. "The Epidemiology of Illness Behavior and Its Relationship to Physical and Psychological Distress," *Symptoms, Illness Behavior, and Help-Seeking*, edited by David Mechanic, Ph.D. Prodist, 1982.

Parkes, C. et al. "Broken Heart: A Statistical Study of Increased Mortality Among Widowers," *British Medical Journal*, Vol. 4, 13–16, 1979.

Pitman, Roger K., Orr, Scott, van der Kolk, Bessel, and Greenberg, Mark. Paper presented at the Annual Meeting of the American Psychiatric Association, Montreal, 1988.

Pitman, Roger K. et al. "Psychophysiologic Assessment of Posttraumatic Stress Disorder Imagery in Vietnam Combat Veterans," *Arch. Gen. Psychiatry*, Vol. 44, November 1987.

Scrignar, C. B., M.D. *Posttraumatic Stress Disorder: Diagnosis, Treatment, and Legal Issues*, Praeger, 1984.

Shore, James H., M.D., *Disaster Stress Studies: New Methods and Studies*. Shore, J. H., ed. Washington, D.C., American Psychiatric Press, 1986.

Shore, James H., M.D., Tatum, Ellie L., M.S.W., and Vollmer, William M., Ph.D. "Psychiatric Reactions to Disaster: The Mount Saint Helens Experience." *American Journal of Psychiatry*, 143: 590–95, 1986.

Shore, James H., M.D., Tatum, Ellie L., M.S.W., and Vollmer, William M., Ph.D. "Evaluation of Mental Health Effects of Disaster: The Mount Saint Helens Eruptions." *American Journal of Public Health*, 76: 76–83 (March suppl.), 1986.

Spiegel, David, M.D.; Hunt, Thurman, B.S.; and Dondershine, Harvey E., M.D., J.D. "Dissociation and Hypnotizability in Posttraumatic Stress Disorder," *American Journal of Psychiatry*, Vol. 143, No. 3, March 1988.

Tennant, Christopher. "Psychosocial Stress and Ischaemic Heart Disease: An Evaluation in the Light of the Diseases' Attribution to War Service," *Australian and New Zealand Journal of Psychiatry*, No. 16, 31–26, 1982.

Trubo, Richard. "Stress and Disease: Cellular Evidence Hints at Therapy," *Medical World News*, January 26, 1987.

Van der Kolk, Bessel A., M.D. "The Drug Treatment of Posttraumatic Stress Disorder," *Journal of Affective Disorders*, No. 13, 203–13, 1987.

———. "Trauma and Chronic Anxiety," *The Psychiatric Times*, 31–32, January 1988.

Zborowski, M. "Cultural Components in Response to Pain." *J Soc Iss*, Vol. 8, 16–30, 1952.

5. WHO IS AT RISK?

Crowe, R. R. et al. "A Family Study of Anxiety Neurosis." *Arch Gen Psychiatry*, Vol. 37, 77–79, 1980.

Dohrenwend, Barbara Snell and Dohrenwend, Bruce P., editors. *Stressful Life Events and Their Contexts*, Prodist, 1981.

Helzer, John E., M.D.; Robins, Lee N., Ph.D.; and McEvoy, Larry, M.A. "Posttraumatic Stress Disorder in the General Population: Findings of the Epidemiologic Catchment Area Survey," *The New England Journal of Medicine*, December 24, 1987.

Horowitz, Mardi J., M.D. "Stress-Response Syndromes: A Review of Posttraumatic and Adjustment Disorders," *Hospital and Community Psychiatry*, Vol. 37, No. 3, March 1986.

McInnes, R. G. "Observations on Hereditary in Neurosis," *Proc R Soc Med;* Vol. 30, 895–904.

Riccelli, Carlene, M.Ed., Ed.D. "Adult Children of Alcoholics on Campus: Programming for a Population at Risk," *JACH*, Vol. 36, September 1987.

Scrignar, C. B., M.D. *Posttraumatic Stress Disorder: Diagnosis, Treatment, and Legal Issues*, Praeger, 1984

6. EVENTS THAT CAN SHAKE YOUR WORLD

American Psychiatric Association: *Diagnostic and Statistical Manual of Mental Disorders*, Third Edition, Revised, Washington, D.C., American Psychiatric Association, 1987.

7. CRIMES AGAINST NATURE: WAR AND VIOLENCE

Allen, Irving M., M.D. "Posttraumatic Stress Disorder Among Black Vietnam Veterans," *Hospital and Community Psychiatry*, Vol. 37, No. 1, January 1986.

Baum, Andrew. "Disasters, Natural and Otherwise," *Psychology Today*, April 1988.

Horn, J. C. "Reactions to Radon," *Psychology Today*, April 1988.

Belenky, Gregory Lucas, M.D. "Psychiatric Casualties: The Israeli Experience," *Psychiatric Annals*, Volume 17, No. 8, August 1987.

Bishop, Katherine. "Veteran Whose Legs Were Severed Is Sued," *The New York Times*, January 24, 1988.

English, Bella. "All That Keeps Him Going," *The Boston Globe*, March 21, 1988.

Gleser, G. C., et al. "Prolonged Psychosocial Effects of Disaster: A Study of Buffalo Creek," Academic Press, 1981.

Greenberg, Keith. "Doctor, Van Take to Streets to Help NYC's Homeless Kids," *USA Today*, December 11, 1987.

Heron, Kim. "The Long Road Back," *The New York Times Magazine*, March 6, 1988.

Hohensemser, C. and Renn, O. "Shifting Public Perceptions of Nuclear Risk: Chernobyl's Other Legacy," *Environment*, Vol. 30, No. 2, April 1988.

Kelly, William E., M.D., editor. *Posttraumatic Stress Disorder and the War Veteran Patient*, Brunner/Mazel, Inc. 1985.

Lerer, Bernard, M.D.; Bleich, Avraham, M.D.; Kotler, Moshe, M.D.; Garb, Ronald, DPM, FF Psych.; Hertzberg, Maya, M.A.; and Levin, Bina. "Posttraumatic Stress Disorder in Israeli Combat Veterans: Effect of Phenelzine Treatment," *Arch. Gen. Psychiatry*, Vol. 44, November 1987.

Lindemann, Erich, M.D. "Symptomatology and Management of Acute Grief," *American Journal of Psychiatry*, Vol. 101: 141–48, 1944.

McFarlane, Alexander Cowell, M.B., B.S., F.R.A.N.Z.C.P. "The Phenomenology of Posttraumatic Stress Disorders following a Natural Disaster," *The Journal of Nervous and Mental Disease*, Vol. 176, No. 1. (Copyright 1988 by The Williams & Wilkins Co.)

McMurran, Kristin. "Facing the Demon: Tireless in His Desperate Cause, a Committed Doctor Battles a Plague," *People Magazine*, April 18, 1988.

Marciniak, Richard D., Cpt., Medical Corps., USAR. "Implications to Forensic Psychiatry of Posttraumatic Stress Disorder: A Review," *Military Medicine*, Vol. 151, August 1986.

Read, P. P. *Alive!*, J. P. Lippincott, 1974.

"Consultation Efforts Following Plane Crash," *Psychiatry '87*, August 1987.

"Teens in the Nuclear Age: Their View of the Future," (Interview with Dr. Eric S. Chivian right after a symposium at the American Psychiatric Association annual meeting in Chicago regarding a survey he and his colleagues did in 1986 of 9,000 U.S., USSR, Swedish, and New Zealand teenagers . . .) *Psychiatry '87*, August 1987.

Pelton, Charles. "Searchers Try to View Task with 'Detachment'," *USA Today*, December 11, 1987.

Scrignar, C. B., M.D. *Posttraumatic Stress Disorder: Diagnosis, Treatment, and Legal Issues*, Praeger, 1984.

Shenson, Douglas, M.D. "When Fear Conquers: A Doctor Learns About AIDS From Leprosy," *The New York Times Magazine*, February 28, 1988.

Shore, James H., M.D., *Disaster Stress Studies: New Methods and Studies*. Shore, J. H., ed. Washington, D.C.: American Psychiatric Press, 1986.

Shore, James H., M.D., Tatum, Ellie L., M.S.W., and Vollmer, William M., Ph.D. "Psychiatric Reactions to Disaster: The Mount Saint Helens Experience." *American Journal of Psychiatry*. 143: 590–95, 1986.

Shore, James H., M.D., Tatum, Ellie L., M.S.W., and Vollmer, William M., Ph.D. "Evaluation of Mental Health Effects of Disaster: The Mount Saint Helens Eruptions." *American Journal of Public Health*, 76: 76–83 (March suppl.), 1986.

Silverman, Joel J. "Posttraumatic Stress Disorder," *Adv. Psychosom. Med.*, Vol. 16, 115–140, Karger, Basel, 1986.

State vs. Marks: Pacific Reporter 647 (2nd series): 1982.

Terr, L. C. "Psychic Trauma in Children: Observations Following Church and School Bus Kidnapping," *American Journal of Psychiatry*, Vol. 138, 14–19, 1981.

8. CRIMES OF THE HEART: PERSONAL AND SOCIAL

Anderson, Craig L., M.S.W. "Males as Sexual Assault Victims: Multiple Levels of Trauma," 145–162, The Haworth Press, Inc., 1982.

Bauer, Anne C. "Emotional Disorders Among Doctors Prompt Programs to Treat Them," *The New York Times*, May 19, 1981.

Begley, Sharon; Murr, Andrew; Springer, Karen; Gordon, Jeanne; Harrison, Joanne; and bureau reports. "All About Twins." *Newsweek*, November 23, 1987.

Brody, Jane E. "Divorce's Stress Exacts Long-Term Health Toll," *The New York Times*, December 13, 1983.

Brown, Murray A., M.D. "A Behavioral Approach to Postcatastrophic Illness Work Phobias," *International Journal of Psychiatry in Medicine*, Vol. 8, No. 3, 1977–78.

Chu, Daniel and Johnson, Bonnie; with Armstrong, Lois; Ash, Jennifer; and Gold, Todd. "Breaking the Bond of Silence," *People Magazine*, April 18, 1988.

Dickens, Monica. "Miracles of Courage," *Reader's Digest*, (Condensed from book of same name, Dodd, Mead, 1985.)

Ginsberg, Susannah and Brown, George W. "No Time for Depression: A Study of Help-Seeking Among Mothers of Preschool Children," *Symptoms, Illness Behavior, and Help-Seeking* edited by David Mechanic, Prodist, 1982.

Goleman, D. "Finding the Right Psychotherapist," *Town and Country*, March 1988.

Goleman, D. "Study of Normal Mourning Process Illuminates Grief Gone Awry," *The New York Times*, March 29, 1988.

Hayes, David N., M.A. "A Description of a Group For Those Who Witness or Discover Suicide," Baton Rouge Crisis Intervention Center, in print.

Kaplan, David M., M.S. and Mason, Edward A., M.D. "Maternal Reactions to Premature Birth Viewed as an Acute Emotional Disorder," *American Journal of Orthopsychiatry*, Vol. 30, 539–547, 1960.

Kobasa, Suzanne Ouellette, Ph.D. "How Much Stress Can You Survive?" *American Health*, September 1984.

Lindemann, Erich, M.D. "Symptomatology and Management of Acute Grief," *American Journal of Psychiatry*, Vol. 101, 141–148, 1944.

Livingston, Dodie Truman, Commissioner, Administration for Children, Youth, and Families, Department of Health and Human Services. "Foreword," *Report of the National Conference on Youth Suicide*, Washington, D.C., June 19–20, 1985.

Mendelson, George. "The Concept of Posttraumatic Stress Disorder: A Review," *International Journal of Law and Psychiatry*, Vol. 10, 45–62, 1987.

Miller, Alice. *The Drama of the Gifted Child*, (Formerly called "A Prisoner of Childhood"), Basic Books, 1983.

Miller, Annetta; with Springen, Karen; Gordon, Jeanne; Murr, Andrew; Cohn, Bob; Drew, Lisa; and Barrett, Todd, "Stress on the Job," *Newsweek*, April 25, 1988.

Moore, David Leon. "Bias' Death Unraveled Coach's Life," *USA Today*, June 8, 1987.

"I Just Didn't Think It Was Any of My Business," Editorial, *Glamour Magazine*, May 1988.

"Predictors of Suicide," *Psychiatry '87*, August 1987.

Rapoport, Rhona, Ph.D. "Normal Crises, Family Structure, and Mental Health," *Family Process*, Vol. 2, 68–80, 1963.

Raymond, Margaret Elmendorf, M.S.W.; Slaby, Andrew Edmund, M.D., M.P.H.; and Lieb, Julian, M.D. *The Healing Alliance*, W. W. Norton & Company, Inc., 1975.

Ross, Charlotte P., President/Executive Director, Youth Suicide National Center. "Foreword," *National Conference on Youth Suicide*, Washington, D.C., June 19–20, 1985.

Rothberg, Joseph M., Ph.D.; Ursano, Robert J., M.D.; and Holloway, Harry C., M.D. "Suicide in the United States Military," *Psychiatric Annals*, Vol. 17, No. 8, August 1987.

Scrignar, C. B., M.D. *Posttraumatic Stress Disorder: Diagnosis, Treatment, and Legal Issues*, Praeger, 1984.

Siwolop, Sana; with Rhein, Reginald, Jr. and Weber, Joe. "The Crippling Ills That Stress Can Trigger," *Business Week*, April 18, 1988.

Slaby, Andrew E., M.D., Ph.D., Glicksman, Arvin S., M.D. *Adapting to Life-Threatening Illness*, Praeger, 1985.

Winerip, Michael. "Where the Rich Find Comfort in Each Other," *The New York Times*, March 1, 1988.

9. CRIMES IN THE FAST TRACK: THE BUSINESS WORLD

Antilla, Susan. "Merger Traumatizes E. F. Hutton Workers," *USA Today*, December 21, 1987.

Bauer, Anne C. "Emotional Disorders Among Doctors Prompt Programs to Treat Them," *The New York Times*, May 19, 1981.

Bolles, Richard Nelson. *What Color is Your Parachute?*, Ten Speed Press, 1984.

Briles, Judith. *Women to Women: From Sabotage to Support*, Far Hills, N.J.: New Horizons Press, 1987.

Calano, J. and Salzman, J. *Career Tracking: How to Get More Done in a Day*. Simon & Schuster, 1987.

Deal, Terrence and Kennedy, Allen. *Corporate Cultures*, Addison-Wesley, 1982.

Deutsch, Claudia H. "Why Being Fired is Losing Its Taint," *The New York Times*, January 24, 1988.

Freudenheim, Milt. "Coping With Stress at Work," *The New York Times*, May 26, 1987.

Kobasa, Suzanne Ouellette, Ph.D. "How Much Stress Can You Survive?" *American Health*, September 1984.

McCormick, John and Powell, Bill. "Management for the 1990s," *Newsweek*, April 25, 1988.

Miller, Annetta; Springen, Karen; Gordon, Jeanne; Murr, Andrew; Cohn, Bob; Drew, Lisa; and Barrett, Todd. "Stress on the Job," *Newsweek*, April 25, 1988.

Myers, A. and Andersen, C. P. *Success Over 60*, Summit, 1984.

Peters, Thomas and Waterman, Robert. *In Search of Excellence*, Warner Books, 1984.

Plumez, Jacqueline Hornor with Dougherty, Karla. *Divorcing a Corporation*, Villard Books, 1986.

Ryan, Michael. "The Yuppies of Wall Street After the Crash," *Glamour Magazine*, May 1988.

Siwolop, Sana; with Rhein, Reginald, Jr. and Weber, Joe. "The Crippling Ills That Stress Can Trigger," *Business Week*, April 18, 1988.

Smith, Emily T.; with Brott, Jody; Cuneo, Alice; and Davis, Jo Ellen. "Stress: The Test Americans are Failing," *Business Week*, April 18, 1988.

Solomon, H. and Chilnick, L. *Beat the Odds*, Villard Books, New York, 1987.

Waggoner, Dianna. "Author Judith Briles Discovers That Women at Work May Be Women at War—Usually with Each Other." *People*, April 18, 1988.

10. A BETTER LIFE IS WAITING

Ettedgui, Eva, M.D. and Bridges, Mary, M.D. "Posttraumatic Stress Disorder," *Psychiatric Clinics of North America*, Vol. 8, No. 1, March 1985.

Horowitz, Mardi J., M.D. "Stress-Response Syndromes: A Review of Posttraumatic and Adjustment Disorders," *Hospital and Community Psychiatry*, Vol. 37, No. 3, March 1986.

Kobasa, Suzanne Ouellette, Ph.D. "How Much Stress Can You Survive?" *American Health*, September 1984.

Maslow, Abraham. *Toward a Psychology of Being*, Princeton: Van Nostrand, 1968.

Slaby, Andrew E. "Crisis-Oriented Therapy," from F. R. Lipton and S. M. Goldfinger's "Emergency Psychiatry at the Crossroads," *New Directions for Mental Health Services*, No. 28, Jossey-Bass, December 1985.

Slaby, Andrew Edmund, M.D., Ph.D., M.P.H., Lieb, Julian, M.D., Tancredi, L. R., M.D., J.D. *The Handbook of Psychiatric Emergency*, Third Edition, Medical Examination Publishing Co., 1985.

Van der Kolk, Bessel A., M.D. "Trauma and Chronic Anxiety," *The Psychiatric Times*, 31–32, January 1988.

11. GOOD NEWS ABOUT MEDICINE

Berlant, Jeffrey L., M.D., Ph.D.; Extein, Irl, M.D.; and Kirstein, Larry S., M.D. *Guide to the New Medicines of the Mind*, The P.I.A. Press, 1988.

Bootzin, Richard R. and Acocella, Joan Ross. *Abnormal Psychology*, Fifth Edition, Random House, 1988. (Chapter 21: "Approaches to Treatment: Biological Therapy, Group Therapy, and Community-Based Services.)

Ettedgui, Eva, M.D. and Bridges, Mary, M.D. "Posttraumatic Stress Disorder," *Psychiatric Clinics of North America*, Vol. 8, No. 1, March 1985.

Falcon, Spencer, M.D.; Ryan, Colleen, M.D.; Chamberlain, Kenneth, M.D.; and Curtis, George, M.D. "Tricyclics: Possible Treatment for Posttraumatic Stress Disorder," *Journal of Clinical Psychiatry*, Vol. 46, 385–389, 1985.

Gerner, Robert H., M.D. "Pharmacological Treatment of Anxiety Disorders," *Psychopharmacology Consultation*, David C. Jimerson, M.D., and John P. Docherty, M.D., eds., American Psychiatric Press, Inc., 1986.

Gold, Mark S., M.D. *The Good News About Depression*, Villard Books, 1987.

Jimerson, David C., M.D. and Docherty, John P., M.D., eds. *Psychopharmacology Consultation*, American Psychiatric Press, Inc., 1986.

Silverman, Joel J. "Posttraumatic Stress Disorder," *Adv. Psychosom. Med.* Vol. 16, 115–140, Karger, Basel, 1986.

Van der Kolk, Bessel A. "The Drug Treatment of Posttraumatic Stress Disorder," *Journal of Affective Disorders*, No. 13, 203–213, 1987.

———. "Psychopharmacological Issues in Posttraumatic Stress Disorder," *Hospital and Community Psychiatry*, Vol. 34, No. 8, August 1983.

12. THERAPY THAT REALLY WORKS

Bedrosian, R. C. and Beck, A. T. *Principles of Cognitive Therapy in Psychotherapy Process: Current Issues and Future Directions*, M. J. Mahoney, ed., Plenum, 1980.

Bootzin, Richard R. and Acocella, Joan Ross. *Abnormal Psychology*, Fifth Edition, Random House, 1988.

Burns, David D., M.D. *Feeling Good: The New Mood Therapy*, William Morrow and Company, Inc., 1980.

Falloon, I. R. H., et al. "Family Management in the Prevention of Morbidity of Schizophrenia," *Arch. Gen. Psychiatry*, Vol. 42, 887–96, 1985.

————. "Family Management in Prevention of Exacerbation of Schizophrenia: A Controlled Study," *The New England Journal of Medicine*, Vol. 306, No. 24, 1437–40, 1982.

Gold, Mark S., M.D. *The Good News About Depression*, Villard Books, 1987.

Raymond, Margaret Elmendorf, M.S.W.; Slaby, Andrew Edmund, M.D., M.P.H.; and Lieb, Julian, M.D. *The Healing Alliance*, W. W. Norton & Company, Inc., 1975.

Scrignar, C. B., M.D. *Post-Traumatic Stress Disorder: Diagnosis, Treatment, and Legal Issues*, Praeger, 1984.

Sloane, R. B., et al. *Psychoanalysis Versus Behavioral Therapy*, Harvard University Press, 1975.

Williams, W. Vail and Polak, Paul R. "Follow-Up Research in Primary Prevention: A Model of Adjustment in Acute Grief," *Journal of Clinical Psychology*, Vol. 35, No. 1, January 1979.

Wolberg, L. *The Technique of Psychotherapy*, Grune & Stratton, Inc., 1977.

13. AN OUNCE OF PREVENTION

Kobasa, Suzanne Ouellette, Ph.D. "How Much Stress Can You Survive?" *American Health*, September 1984.

Slaby, Andrew E., M.D., Ph.D., M.P.H. *Sixty Ways to Make Stress Work for You*, The P.I.A. Press, 1988.

Slaby, Andrew E., M.D., Ph.D., and Glicksman, Arvin S., M.D. *Adapting to Life-Threatening Illness*, Praeger, 1985.

Solomon, Harold S., M.D., and Chilnick, Lawrence D. *Beat the Odds*, The P.I.A. Press, Villard Books, 1987.

14. STOPPING STRESS STEP-BY-STEP

Jeffers, Susan, Ph.D. *Feel the Fear and Do it Anyway*, Harcourt Brace Jovanovich, 1987.

Perlmutter, Cathy. "Comic Relief," *Prevention*, March 1988.

Slaby, Andrew E., M.D., Ph.D., M.P.H. *Sixty Ways to Make Stress Work for You*, The P.I.A. Press, 1988.

———. *Beat the Odds*, P.I.A. Press, Villard Books, 1987.

EPILOGUE: WELCOME, CRISIS

Slaby, Andrew E. "Crisis-Oriented Therapy," from F. R. Lipton and S. M. Goldfinger's "Emergency Psychiatry at the Crossroads," *New Directions for Mental Health Services*, No. 28, Jossey-Bass, December 1985.

———. *Sixty Ways to Make Stress Work for You*, The P.I.A. Press, 1988.

OTHER RESOURCES

For information on evaluation and treatment, contact:

Andrew E. Slaby, M.D., Ph.D., M.P.H.
Fair Oaks Hospital
19 Prospect Street
Summit, N.J. 07901
1 800-HELPLINE

For additional information, you may contact:

National Organization for Victim Assistance
717 D Street, N.W.
Suite 200
Washington, D.C. 20004
1 202 393-NOVA

Vietnam Veterans of America
2001 S Street, N.W.
Washington, D.C. 20009
1 202 332-2700

Veterans Administration
810 Vermont Avenue, N.W.
Washington D.C. 20420
1 202 233-4000

INDEX

ABOUT THE AUTHOR

ANDREW E. SLABY, M.D., PH.D., M.P.H., is a nationally prominent epidemiologist, psychiatrist, and specialist in human behavior. Medical Director of Fair Oaks Hospital, Summit, New Jersey, Dr. Slaby is also Adjunct Professor of Psychiatry and Human Behavior at Brown University and Clinical Professor of Psychiatry at New York University and The New York Medical College. Dr. Slaby is the author of numerous scientific books, papers, and research studies. Frequently appearing on television and radio programs as an expert, Dr. Slaby lectures on personal crisis intervention/management, depression, suicide prevention, management of violent individuals, and techniques people can use to adapt to life-threatening stress or illness. He also writes and lectures on the management of stress in adolescents and college-age individuals. The recipient of many scientific prizes and awards, Dr. Slaby is a graduate of the Columbia University's College of Physicians and Surgeons and of Yale University.